OTHER FAST FACTS BOOKS

Fast Facts About PTSD: A Guide for Nurses and Other Health Care Professionals (*Adams*)

Fast Facts for the NEW NURSE PRACTITIONER: What You Really Need to Know in a Nutshell, Second Edition (*Aktan*)

Fast Facts for the ER NURSE: Emergency Department Orientation in a Nutshell, Third Edition (*Buettner*)

Fast Facts About GI AND LIVER DISEASES FOR NURSES: What APRNs Need to Know in a Nutshell (*Chaney*)

Fast Facts for the MEDICAL–SURGICAL NURSE: Clinical Orientation in a Nutshell (*Ciocco*)

Fast Facts on COMBATING NURSE BULLYING, INCIVILITY, AND WORKPLACE VIOLENCE: What Nurses Need to Know in a Nutshell (*Ciocco*)

Fast Facts for the NURSE PRECEPTOR: Keys to Providing a Successful Preceptorship in a Nutshell (*Ciocco*)

Fast Facts for the OPERATING ROOM NURSE: An Orientation and Care Guide, Second Edition (*Criscitelli*)

Fast Facts for the ANTEPARTUM AND POSTPARTUM NURSE: A Nursing Orientation and Care Guide in a Nutshell (*Davidson*)

Fast Facts for the NEONATAL NURSE: A Nursing Orientation and Care Guide in a Nutshell (*Davidson*)

Fast Facts Workbook for CARDIAC DYSRHYTHMIAS AND 12-LEAD EKGs (*Desmarais*)

Fast Facts About PRESSURE ULCER CARE FOR NURSES: How to Prevent, Detect, and Resolve Them in a Nutshell (*Dziedzic*)

Fast Facts for the GERONTOLOGY NURSE: A Nursing Care Guide in a Nutshell (*Eliopoulos*)

Fast Facts for the LONG-TERM CARE NURSE: What Nursing Home and Assisted Living Nurses Need to Know in a Nutshell (*Eliopoulos*)

Fast Facts for the CLINICAL NURSE MANAGER: Managing a Changing Workplace in a Nutshell, Second Edition (*Fry*)

Fast Facts for EVIDENCE-BASED PRACTICE IN NURSING: Implementing EBP in a Nutshell, Second Edition (*Godshall*)

Fast Facts for Nurses About HOME INFUSION THERAPY: The Expert's Best Practice Guide in a Nutshell (*Gorski*)

Fast Facts About NURSING AND THE LAW: Law for Nurses in a Nutshell (*Grant, Ballard*)

Fast Facts for the L&D NURSE: Labor & Delivery Orientation in a Nutshell, Second Edition (*Groll*)

Fast Facts for the RADIOLOGY NURSE: An Orientation and Nursing Care Guide in a Nutshell (*Grossman*)

Fast Facts on ADOLESCENT HEALTH FOR NURSING AND HEALTH PROFESSIONALS: A Care Guide in a Nutshell (*Herrman*)

Fast Facts for the FAITH COMMUNITY NURSE: Implementing FCN/Parish Nursing in a Nutshell (*Hickman*)

Fast Facts for the CARDIAC SURGERY NURSE: Caring for Cardiac Surgery Patients in a Nutshell, Second Edition (*Hodge*)

Fast Facts About the NURSING PROFESSION: Historical Perspectives in a Nutshell (*Hunt*)

Fast Facts for the CLINICAL NURSING INSTRUCTOR: Clinical Teaching in a Nutshell, Third Edition (*Kan, Stabler-Haas*)

Fast Facts for the WOUND CARE NURSE: Practical Wound Management in a Nutshell (*Kifer*)

Fast Facts About EKGs FOR NURSES: The Rules of Identifying EKGs in a Nutshell (*Landrum*)

Fast Facts for the CRITICAL CARE NURSE: Critical Care Nursing in a Nutshell (*Landrum*)

Fast Facts for the TRAVEL NURSE: Travel Nursing in a Nutshell (*Landrum*)

Fast Facts for the SCHOOL NURSE: School Nursing in a Nutshell, Second Edition (*Loschiavo*)

Fast Facts for MANAGING PATIENTS WITH A PSYCHIATRIC DISORDER: What RNs, NPs, and New Psych Nurses Need to Know (*Marshall*)

Fast Facts About SUBSTANCE USE DISORDERS: What Every Nurse, APRN, and PA Needs to Know (*Marshall, Spencer*)

Fast Facts About CURRICULUM DEVELOPMENT IN NURSING: How to Develop and Evaluate Educational Programs in a Nutshell, Second Edition (*McCoy, Anema*)

Fast Facts for the CATH LAB NURSE (*McCulloch*)

Fast Facts About NEUROCRITICAL CARE: A Quick Reference for the Advanced Practice Provider (*McLaughlin*)

Fast Facts for DEMENTIA CARE: What Nurses Need to Know in a Nutshell (*Miller*)

Fast Facts for HEALTH PROMOTION IN NURSING: Promoting Wellness in a Nutshell (*Miller*)

Fast Facts for STROKE CARE NURSING: An Expert Care Guide, Second Edition (*Morrison*)

Fast Facts for the MEDICAL OFFICE NURSE: What You Really Need to Know in a Nutshell (*Richmeier*)

Fast Facts for the PEDIATRIC NURSE: An Orientation Guide in a Nutshell (*Rupert, Young*)

Fast Facts About FORENSIC NURSING: What You Need to Know (*Scannell*)

Fast Facts About the GYNECOLOGICAL EXAM: A Professional Guide for NPs, PAs, and Midwives, Second Edition (*Secor, Fantasia*)

Fast Facts for the STUDENT NURSE: Nursing Student Success in a Nutshell (*Stabler-Haas*)

Fast Facts for CAREER SUCCESS IN NURSING: Making the Most of Mentoring in a Nutshell (*Vance*)

Fast Facts for the TRIAGE NURSE: An Orientation and Care Guide, Second Edition (*Visser, Montejano*)

Fast Facts for DEVELOPING A NURSING ACADEMIC PORTFOLIO: What You Really Need to Know in a Nutshell (*Wittmann-Price*)

Fast Facts for the HOSPICE NURSE: A Concise Guide to End-of-Life Care (*Wright*)

Fast Facts for the CLASSROOM NURSING INSTRUCTOR: Classroom Teaching in a Nutshell (*Yoder-Wise, Kowalski*)

Forthcoming FAST FACTS Books

Fast Facts About NEUROPATHIC PAIN (*Davies*)

Fact Facts in HEALTH INFORMATICS FOR NURSES (*Hardy*)

Fact Facts About NURSE ANESTHESIA (*Hickman*)

Fast Facts for the CARDIAC SURGERY NURSE, Third Edition (*Hodge*)

Fast Facts for the CRITICAL CARE NURSE: Critical Care Nursing, Second Edition (*Landrum*)

Fast Facts for the SCHOOL NURSE, Third Edition (*Loschiavo*)

Fast Facts on How to Conduct, Understand, and Maybe Even Love RESEARCH! For Nurses and Other Healthcare Providers (*Marshall*)

Fast Facts About RELIGION FOR NURSES: Implications for Patient Care (*Taylor*)

Visit www.springerpub.com to order.

FAST FACTS for
THE TRIAGE NURSE

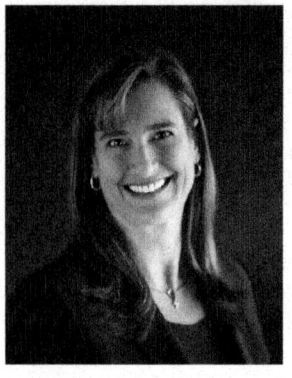

Lynn Sayre Visser, MSN, RN, PHN, CEN, CPEN, is a registered nurse and award-winning author with nearly 30 years of experience in emergency nursing and prehospital care. She holds national certifications in emergency nursing and pediatric emergency nursing. Her passion for triage led to instrumental roles in teaching formalized triage education, orienting nurses to triage, and improving throughput processes. She is the author of the pocket-sized chief complaint–based book *Rapid Access Guide for Triage and Emergency Nurses: Chief Complaints With High Risk Presentations* and the first edition of *Fast Facts for the Triage Nurse: An Orientation and Care Guide in a Nutshell*, which won third place in the 2015 *American Journal of Nursing* Book of the Year Awards in the critical care/emergency category. She has touched the nursing profession on a global level with the Fast Facts book now available internationally under the title *Essentials for the Triage Nurse: An Orientation and Care Guide in a Nutshell*. She has been recognized by her peers for her triage work and contributions to emergency nursing with a nomination for the Emergency Nurses Association (ENA) Distinguished Certified Emergency Nurse Award as well as the ENA Team Award.

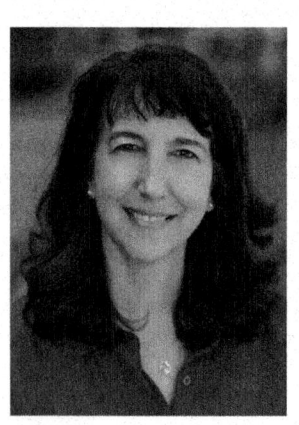

Anna Sivo Montejano, DNP, RN, PHN, CEN, has 33 years of experience in nursing with a specialty in emergency and triage education. She has taught nursing theory and aided the professional development of nurses as a preceptor, mentor, and clinical instructor. She has been a certified emergency nurse for more than 25 years. Her ED contributions include work as a staff nurse, primary preceptor, and assistant nurse manager as well as in educational development. Dr. Montejano has worked to improve the quality and efficiency of patient care through projects such as the change process of rapid medical screenings and rapid triage assessments, as a project manager for a major ED expansion, and as an advanced cardiac life support instructor. She coauthored "What Is a Triage Nurse?" published in the *Journal of Emergency Nursing*. She is the recipient of a nomination for the Emergency Nurses Association Team Award for her involvement with improvements in triage processes and received third place in the

One of the things that draws nurses into the specialty of emergency nursing is that we love environments where things happen quickly and we are often drawn to brevity. I cannot think of a better format for emergency nurses to learn about the challenges of triage than a book that presents the facts in such a concise and consolidated fashion. It serves as an excellent resource for all emergency nurses, written by respected names in the emergency world.

Jeff Solheim, MSN, RN, CEN, CFRN, TCRN, FAEN, FAAN
President
Solheim Enterprises

A concise yet comprehensive reference that cuts to the chase, just like a good emergency nurse. With content covering hot topics such as active shooter situations, pain management, and human trafficking, this book has something for triage nurses at all stages of the novice-to-expert continuum.

Jean A. Proehl, RN, MN, CEN, CPEN, TCRN, FAEN, FAAN
Emergency Clinical Nurse Specialist, Proehl PRN, LLC
Education Director & Team Leader, Project Helping Hands

A dream team of authors, contributors, and reviewers created a one-of-a-kind masterpiece on triage nursing. Building upon the invaluable first edition content, the second edition adds more chapters to cover current nursing concerns. Nurses with various experience levels and practicing in any field will certainly benefit from this easy-to-read and easy-to-understand book. A must-have for every nurse's personal library!

Donna Wilk Cardillo, RN, CSP, FAAN
The Inspiration Nurse and author of The ULTIMATE Career Guide for Nurses: Practical Advice for Thriving at Every Stage of Your Career and Falling Together: How to Find Balance, Joy, and Meaningful Change When Your Life Seems to Be Falling Apart

A gem of a book, straight to the point with a wealth of knowledge in a nutshell. This condensed, compact, and comprehensive quick resource zeroes in on all the essentials of triage nursing. Clear and concise, this book is a must for all emergency department nurses.

Laura Gasparis Vonfrolio, PhD, RN
CEO of www.GreatNurses.com

An easy-to-read guide living up to its claim of providing information "in a nutshell." The editors have drawn subject matter experts from across the Emergency Nursing profession to write on topics spanning emergency triage tips and regulatory elements through complaint-specific chapters. The book is formatted in bullet points to get right to answering questions for the Emergency Triage Nurse without extra fluff. "Red flags" sections in the chapters help readers zero in on patient safety and quality care while building Emergency Triage Nurse confidence. This resource WILL become part of your valued Emergency Nurse library.

Andi Foley, DNP, RN, ACCNS-AG, CEN
Emergency Services CNS
"Triage Decisions" section editor for the Journal of Emergency Nursing

For your novice nurse to your most tenured nurse in the department. This book truly has something for everyone in the ED, not only the triage the nurse. The chapters are broken down so, no matter your expertise level, you can understand what is being presented and learn to provide the best care possible for your patients.

Mike Hastings, MSN, RN, CEN
Clinical Manager Emergency Department

An incredible resource for any emergency department nurse. Information is concise and well organized for quick reference. Topics are very practical and can be applied to your very next shift. If you're new to emergency nursing, this book is a must-have!

Kati Kleber, MSN, RN, CCRN-K
Author, nurse, and creator of the FreshRN® website

Fast Facts for the Triage Nurse: An Orientation and Care Guide is just that! It is a concise, user-friendly orientation guide and reference manual for many members of the healthcare team—nurses, prehospital providers, educators, preceptors, and frankly anyone who provides care at triage. This comprehensive book offers key concepts that providers will use on a daily basis while working in the triage area. New chapters in the second edition include Triage Competency, Pain Management, Endocrine Emergencies, Disaster, and Active Shooter. There is even a chapter on working with a provider in triage. This book is written by emergency nurses for all emergency care providers. This is a "must-have" to read from cover to cover and it will fit nicely into any lab coat pocket.

K. Sue Hoyt, PhD, RN, FNP-BC, ENP-C, FAEN, FAANP, FAAN
Author of Family Emergent/Urgent and
Ambulatory Care: The Pocket NP

All-inclusive yet rapid-paced reading, great resource for emergency nurses. I especially appreciate the tips for evaluating pediatric and older adults.

Pam D. Bartley, BSN, RN, CEN, CFRN, CPEN, TCRN, CCRN, CTRN
CEO of PDB Nurse Education, LLC

A great concise reference for any triage nurse. The authors have obvious "real world" experience as emergency nurses. It's an easy, readable reference and the "red flags" are tried and true-life patient situations. I would highly recommend this book as it's applicable to both the novice and experienced emergency nurse.

Terry M. Foster, MSN, RN, CEN, CPEN, TCRN, CCRN, FAEN
Critical-Care Clinical Nurse Specialist, Emergency Departments
Saint Elizabeth Healthcare, Edgewood, Kentucky

A thorough, concise, and well-written handbook providing important information for anyone working in the triage arena. A quick read that keeps your attention and delivers down-to-earth, "in the trenches" dialogue with pertinent, friendly advice and examples. Everything that can walk into the triage area is covered in a succinct yet encompassing way. Well done!

Pat Clutter, MEd, RN, CEN, FAEN
ED Staff Nurse Mercy Lebanon
Independent Educator
Journalist

Very impressed by the layout, organization, readability, and up-to-date information in this handy reference. Any triage nurse will be a step ahead by having this practice guide—it's like having a seasoned ED nurse in your pocket at all times. Excellent, excellent!

Beth Hawkes MSN, RN-BC, HACP ("Nurse Beth")
Career Columnist, Writer, Speaker

Not just for nurses. EMS, check this book out! I am a 20+ year paramedic and EMS educator, and I found many of the principles of this book to be very relevant to EMS—a book that works for both hospital and prehospital education.

Lori Gallian, EMT-P
Chief Connector, Summit Sciences

This book is a true gem and takes much of the guesswork out of the RN's triage process. A must-read for all RNs working in the often-overwhelming and chaotic world of emergency nursing!

Thomas Rhodes, BSN, RN, MPA-HSM
Director of Nursing

The authors did an excellent job writing an accurate and up-to-date guide for triage nurses. Fast Facts found within each chapter is invaluable! As a nurse with 23 years of ER and critical care experience, I would like to see a copy of this book on every triage desk!

Laurie Pittman, BSN, RN, CPEN
Staff Nurse

2015 *American Journal of Nursing* Book of the Year Awards, and in the critical care/emergency category for *Fast Facts for the Triage Nurse: An Orientation and Care Guide in a Nutshell*. She recently coauthored *Rapid Access Guide for Triage and Emergency Nurses*.

CONTRIBUTORS

Erik Angle, RN, MICN, MEP Emergency Preparedness Program Coordinator, Sutter Roseville Medical Center, Roseville, California

Shelley Cohen, MSN, RN, CEN Educator/Consultant: Health Resources Unlimited, Staff Nurse: Williamson Medical Center, Franklin, Tennessee

Dawn Friedly Gray, MSN, RN, CEN, CCRN Clinical Coordinator: Emergency Department, Paoli Hospital, Paoli, Pennsylvania

Valerie Aarne Grossman, MALS, BSN, RN, NE-BC Nurse Manager, University of Rochester: Highland Hospital, Rochester, New York

Reneé Semonin Holleran, FNP-BC, PhD, CEN, CCRN (emeritus), CFRN and CTRN (retired), FAEN Nurse Practitioner, Holistic Medicine, Pain Medicine, Veterans Health Administration, Salt Lake City, Utah

Deb Jeffries, MSN-Ed, RN, CEN, CPEN Clinical Education Specialist, Emergency Services, Banner Health, Phoenix, Arizona

Rebecca S. McNair, RN, CEN President/Founder, Triage First, Inc., Veteran Owned Small Business, Fairview, North Carolina

Polly Gerber Zimmermann, MS, MBA, RN-BC, CEN, FAEN Associate Professor, Ivy Tech Community College, Indianapolis, Indiana

FAST FACTS for THE TRIAGE NURSE

An Orientation and Care Guide

Second Edition

Lynn Sayre Visser, MSN, RN, PHN, CEN, CPEN
Anna Sivo Montejano, DNP, RN, PHN, CEN

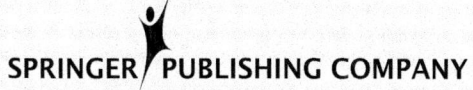

Copyright © 2019 Springer Publishing Company, LLC

All rights reserved.

No part of this publication may be reproduced, stored in a retrieval system, or transmitted in any form or by any means, electronic, mechanical, photocopying, recording, or otherwise, without the prior permission of Springer Publishing Company, LLC, or authorization through payment of the appropriate fees to the Copyright Clearance Center, Inc., 222 Rosewood Drive, Danvers, MA 01923, 978-750-8400, fax 978-646-8600, info@copyright.com or on the Web at www.copyright.com.

Springer Publishing Company, LLC
11 West 42nd Street
New York, NY 10036
www.springerpub.com

Acquisitions Editor: Elizabeth Nieginski
Compositor: Amnet Systems

ISBN: 978-0-8261-4829-2
e-book ISBN: 978-0-8261-4851-3

19 20 21 22 23 / 5 4 3 2 1

The author and the publisher of this Work have made every effort to use sources believed to be reliable to provide information that is accurate and compatible with the standards generally accepted at the time of publication. Because medical science is continually advancing, our knowledge base continues to expand. Therefore, as new information becomes available, changes in procedures become necessary. We recommend that the reader always consult current research and specific institutional policies before performing any clinical procedure. The author and publisher shall not be liable for any special, consequential, or exemplary damages resulting, in whole or in part, from the readers' use of, or reliance on, the information contained in this book. The publisher has no responsibility for the persistence or accuracy of URLs for external or third-party Internet websites referred to in this publication and does not guarantee that any content on such websites is, or will remain, accurate or appropriate.

Library of Congress Cataloging-in-Publication Data

Names: Visser, Lynn Sayre, editor. | Montejano, Anna Sivo, editor.
Title: Fast facts for the triage nurse : an orientation and care guide /
  [edited by] Lynn Sayre Visser, Anna Sivo Montejano.
Description: Second edition. | New York, NY : Springer Publishing Company,
  LLC, [2019] | Series: Fast facts | Includes bibliographical references and
  index.
Identifiers: LCCN 2018039931 (print) | LCCN 2018041089 (ebook) | ISBN
  9780826148513 | ISBN 9780826148292 (print : alk. paper) | ISBN
  9780826148513 (e-book)
Subjects: | MESH: Triage—methods | Emergencies—nursing | Emergency
  Nursing—methods | Emergency Treatment—nursing
Classification: LCC RC86.7 (ebook) | LCC RC86.7 (print) | NLM WY 154.2 | DDC
  616.02/5—dc23
LC record available at https://lccn.loc.gov/2018039931

Contact us to receive discount rates on bulk purchases.
We can also customize our books to meet your needs.
For more information, please contact sales@springerpub.com.

Publisher's Note: New and used products purchased from third-party sellers are not guaranteed for quality, authenticity, or access to any included digital components.

Printed in the United States of America.

To triage nurses everywhere~
Few people can understand what you encounter each shift—the
overwhelming and unpredictable influx of patients,
the sights and sounds of distress, the stories that
simply do not make sense—yet you professionally balance the chaos
with flawless precision, making split-second decisions
in the best interest of each patient.
Your selfless acts, gentle hands, and
compassionate hearts touch the lives of many. Your commitment to
excellence is deserving of a book dedicated to you.

Contents

Reviewers	*xix*
Foreword Rebecca S. McNair, RN, CEN	*xxiii*
Preface	*xxv*
~A Heartfelt Thank You~	*xxvii*
Acknowledgments	*xxix*

Part I SETTING THE STAGE FOR SUCCESS AT TRIAGE

1. **Orienting to Triage** — 3
   Lynn Sayre Visser

2. **Precepting at Triage** — 11
   Lynn Sayre Visser

3. **Tips for Success at Triage** — 21
   Lynn Sayre Visser and Anna Sivo Montejano

4. **Personal Awareness for the Triage Nurse** — 29
   Anna Sivo Montejano

5. **Triage Competency** — 33
   Shelley Cohen

Part II POINT-OF-ENTRY PROCESSES IN TRIAGE NURSING

6. **The Patient Arrival** — 41
   Anna Sivo Montejano

7. **The Patient Experience in Triage Nursing** — 49
   Lynn Sayre Visser

8. **Legal Concerns in Triage Nursing** — 59
Deb Jeffries

Part III NURSING ESSENTIALS FOR EFFECTIVE TRIAGE

9. **Triage Acuity Scales** — 69
Deb Jeffries

10. **Triage Documentation** — 75
Rebecca S. McNair

11. **Time-Sensitive Medical Conditions** — 81
Lynn Sayre Visser

Part IV CURRENT TRENDS IMPACTING TRIAGE NURSING

12. **Urgent Care Triage** — 93
Valerie Aarne Grossman

13. **Electronic Medical Record Considerations** — 97
Dawn Friedly Gray

14. **Provider in Triage** — 101
Lynn Sayre Visser

15. **Advanced Triage Protocols** — 111
Dawn Friedly Gray

Part V "RED FLAG" PATIENT PRESENTATIONS

16. **Introduction to "Red Flag" Presentations** — 119
Lynn Sayre Visser

17. **Respiratory Emergencies** — 125
Polly Gerber Zimmermann and Lynn Sayre Visser

18. **Cardiac Emergencies** — 133
Polly Gerber Zimmermann

19. **Neurological Emergencies** — 139
Reneé Semonin Holleran

20. **Abdominal Emergencies** — 145
Polly Gerber Zimmermann and Lynn Sayre Visser

21. **Obstetric and Gynecological Emergencies** — 153
Lynn Sayre Visser and Polly Gerber Zimmermann

22.	Behavioral Health Emergencies *Anna Sivo Montejano*	161
23.	Ocular Emergencies *Anna Sivo Montejano and Lynn Sayre Visser*	167
24.	Musculoskeletal Emergencies *Reneé Semonin Holleran*	173
25.	Endocrine Emergencies *Dawn Friedly Gray*	177
26.	Environmental Emergencies *Anna Sivo Montejano*	181
27.	Trauma Emergencies *Reneé Semonin Holleran*	187
28.	Infectious Presentations *Anna Sivo Montejano and Lynn Sayre Visser*	193

Part VI SPECIAL CONSIDERATIONS IN TRIAGE NURSING

29.	Special Populations in Triage *Anna Sivo Montejano*	201
30.	Pediatric Triage *Deb Jeffries*	211
31.	Older Adult Triage *Anna Sivo Montejano*	221
32.	Pain Management at Triage *Reneé Semonin Holleran*	229
33.	Patient and Staff Safety *Anna Sivo Montejano*	233
34.	Case Studies in Triage Nursing *Anna Sivo Montejano and Lynn Sayre Visser*	241

Part VII DISASTER SITUATIONS IN TRIAGE NURSING

35.	Emergency Management: A Triage Nurse's Guide for When Disaster Strikes *Erik Angle*	247
36.	Active Shooter or Active Violence *Erik Angle*	255

Abbreviations	263
Appendix A: Resources	267
Appendix B: Triage Competency Validation Form	269
Appendix C: Sample Triage Education and Competency Plan	271
Appendix D: Sample Triage Retrospective Chart Review Audit Form	273
Appendix E: Disaster Triage Tag	275
Additional Reading	279
Index	293

Reviewers

SECOND EDITION

Meredith Addison, MSN, RN, CEN, FAEN
Staff Nurse
Emergency Department
Regional Hospital
Terre Haute, Indiana

Joop Breuer, RN, CEN, FAEN
Nurse Educator/Staff Nurse
Emergency Department
Leiden University Medical Centre
Leiden, The Netherlands

Keith Carlson, BSN, RN, NC-BC
Nurse Career Coach, Podcaster, Author, Speaker
NurseKeith.com
Santa Fe, New Mexico

Teresa Coyne, BSN, RN, CEN
Clinical Coordinator—Staff Nurse
Katy Convenient Care Center, Memorial Hermann (Freestanding ER)
Katy, Texas

Jennifer Denno MSN, RN, CEN, FAEN
Clinical Nurse Educator
Emergency Services
Sutter Medical Center, Sacramento
Sacramento, California

Mary Fardanesh, BSN, RN
Staff Nurse II
Emergency Department
Kaiser Permanente
Roseville, California

Dawn Friedly Gray, MSN, RN, CEN, CCRN
Clinical Coordinator
Emergency Department
Paoli Hospital
Paoli, Pennsylvania

Valerie Aarne Grossman, MALS, BSN, RN, NE-BC
Nurse Manager
University of Rochester: Highland Hospital
Rochester, New York

Reviewers

Steven J. Jewell, BSN, RN, CEN, CPEN, USN (retired)

Critical Care Registered Nurse, GS-11
San Antonio Military Medical Center
Department of Emergency Medicine
Fort Sam Houston, Texas

Larry Masterman, MICP, CEM

Emergency Management/ Homeland Security Consultant
Preparedness Consulting & Training, Int'l.
Weaverville, California

Rebecca S. McNair, RN, CEN

President/Founder, Triage First, Inc.
Veteran Owned Small Business
Fairview, North Carolina

Michelle Michael-Korn, MS, RN, CEN

Director of Nursing, Emergency Services
Samaritan Medical Center
Watertown, New York

Karla Nygren, BSN, RN, CEN, CFRN, CPEN, TCRN, CCRN, CPN

Emergency Department Staff RN/ Patient Care Supervisor
Avera McKennan Hospital and University Health Center
Sioux Falls, South Dakota

Wende M. Ryan, MS, RN-BC, CEN, CCRN

Staff Nurse
Wollongong Hospital
Wollongong, Australia

Nancy Shelton, BSN, RN, EMT-P

Clinical Documentation Specialist
St. Vincent's East
Birmingham, Alabama

Susen Sprowl, BSN, RN, CEN

Staff Nurse, Emergency Services
Sutter Medical Center Sacramento
Sacramento, California

Andrew Wong, MSN, AG-ACNP, RN, CEN, CPEN, CCRN-K

Emergency Department Staff Educator
American Heart Association Training Center Faculty
Department of Emergency Medicine | Department of Nursing Education and Professional Development
Lenox Hill Hospital
Northwell Health System
New York, New York

FIRST EDITION

Meredith Addison, MSN, RN, CEN, FAEN
Staff Nurse
Emergency Department
Regional Hospital
Terre Haute, Indiana

Jessica Castner, PhD, RN, CEN
Assistant Professor
University of Buffalo School of Nursing
Buffalo, New York

Mary Fardanesh, BSN, RN
Staff Nurse 1
Emergency Department
Kaiser Permanente South Sacramento Medical Center
Sacramento, California

Dawn Friedly Gray, MSN, RN, CEN, CCRN
Clinical Coordinator
Emergency Department
Paoli Hospital
Paoli, Pennsylvania

Dawn Hitchcock, MD
Board Certified in Emergency Medicine
California Emergency Physicians
Sutter Roseville Medical Center
Roseville, California

Deb Jeffries, MSN-Ed, RN-BC, CEN, CPEN
Clinical Education Specialist
Banner Desert Medical Center Emergency Department
Cardon Children's Medical Center Emergency Department
Mesa, Arizona

Rebecca S. McNair, RN, CEN
President/Founder, Triage First, Inc.
Veteran Owned Small Business
Fairview, North Carolina

Michelle Michael-Korn, MS, RN, CEN
Director of Nursing, Emergency Services
Samaritan Medical Center
Watertown, New York

Wende M. Ryan, MS, RN-BC, CEN, CCRN
Clinical Educator, Critical Care
Rochester General Health Systems
Rochester, New York

Alexandra Schneider, PhD, PsyD, RN, FNP, LNCC, NY-SAFE
Honeoye Valley Family Practice
University of Rochester School of Nursing
Strong Memorial Hospital Emergency Room
Lima, New York

Nancy Shelton, BSN, RN, EMT-P
Staff Nurse
Emergency Department
St. Vincent's Hospital
Birmingham, Alabama

Andrew Wong, RN, CEN, CPEN
Staff Nurse
Lenox Hill Emergency Department
North Shore Long Island Jewish Health System
Woodside, New York

Foreword

In 2011, the American Nurses Association recognized emergency nursing as a specialty. Within that specialty, areas of focus have been developed to standardize the knowledge and practice base to enable a wide range of practitioners, from novice to expert, to provide excellent evidence-based clinical care across a wide spectrum of healthcare facilities—from small rural to large urban trauma centers. While standardization in some areas has been effected through courses such as the Trauma Nursing Core Course (TNCC), Emergency Nursing Pediatric Course (ENPC), and Advanced Cardiovascular Life Support (ACLS), the art and science of emergency nursing triage has had a longer period of development and standardization. Standardization in this field is critical because correct triage requires a broad knowledge base of *all* these areas as well as excellent decision-making skills and tools.

Lynn Sayre Visser has devoted her career to emergency nursing and triage education, believing each patient deserves unbiased care that is nothing short of excellent. She has a "can-do, never give up, reach for the stars" mindset, which makes her an exemplary nursing role model. She has published in a variety of arenas, was the 2011 Emergency Nurses Association conference blogger, and has been nominated as a Distinguished Certified Emergency Nurse.

Anna Sivo Montejano has a passion for healthcare delivered in the emergency setting. Her intense desire for quality triage, paired with her compelling enthusiasm for the teaching of others, has allowed her to touch lives across the emergency nursing continuum. She is making a difference: from delivering the highest quality patient care, to teaching students, to writing for publication.

Both Lynn Sayre Visser and Anna Sivo Montejano have shown purposeful and energetic devotion to the development of the art and science of emergency triage. Their enthusiasm and dedication to the holistic education of healthcare providers has my utmost admiration, and I consider them to be rising stars in this arena. Among the group of Triage First educators, they consistently stood out as having the most excellent evaluations and have proved themselves worthy of a following.

These authors/editors join together in leading a line of nursing authors, researchers, and teachers of triage to present essential information for the triage nurse to access quickly and repeatedly. *Fast Facts for the Triage Nurse* covers every area of triage in a concise and professional manner, starting with the essentials of triage orientation, preceptorship, competency, and self-care of the triage nurse, and including "Tips for Success at Triage," a chapter created using helpful snippets of triage information from national emergency nursing experts. The book goes on to address point-of-entry processes, nursing essentials, and current trends that impact the initial patient–nurse encounter and are useful in settings from urgent care to the emergency department. Additional sections address "red flag" clinical presentations, special populations, and case studies to help the triage nurse understand these risky areas of triage nursing. The final sections focus on the triage nurse's role if faced with any type of disaster including an active shooter either within or outside the triage area.

The first edition of this book was certainly deserving of its third-place honor in the 2015 *American Journal of Nursing* Book of the Year Awards in the critical care/emergency category. The second edition offers an even greater opportunity to examine and discuss every aspect of triage nursing concepts and skills, including some uncomfortable yet very necessary topics. "Fast Facts" located throughout the book highlight critical information for easy reference. Without hesitation this book will be valuable for anyone practicing triage.

Rebecca S. McNair, RN, CEN
President/Founder, Triage First, Inc.
Fairview, North Carolina

Preface

The purpose of this book is to provide new and seasoned nurses, preceptors, educators, and management teams with foundational skills that can be used throughout the triage orientation process as well as when practicing as an experienced triage nurse. Highlighted concepts include building confidence in the triage role, accurately assessing patient presentations, reducing personnel and hospital liability, increasing patient and staff satisfaction, and, ultimately, delivering quality patient care that supports best outcomes.

Triage is one of the toughest jobs in healthcare. Patients rarely present to triage with a diagnosis, but rather they convey what is often a multitude of complaints, signs, and symptoms that must be weeded through to effectively determine how sick they really are. The authors of this book have years of experience practicing, teaching, and writing about triage to support the reader in the journey toward enhancing triage knowledge.

The main themes and objectives focus on numerous aspects of triage, from front-end processes and orientation to clinical practice and nursing essentials. The diverse factors of patient populations—age, gender, ethnicity, socioeconomic status, and so on—all impact the care a patient receives. A patient may present with a simple laceration, but a self-inflicted wound and a history of mental illness may lead to safety issues for the patient and the individuals in his or her immediate environment. Patient care must be individualized to each patient for each visit. This book details the many aspects of triage in an organized manner using real-life examples to harden the facts.

The book is divided into parts to help organize the flow of information. The establishment of orientation and self-care early on sets the stage for a nurse to be successful in the triage setting. The sections cover workflow and "red flag" presentations, introduced in an organized manner with easy-to-find information. Each chapter contains a brief introduction as well as objectives, followed by "just the facts" information. Content that should not be missed is highlighted in the "Fast Facts" boxes throughout the book. The term *provider* is threaded throughout the content and represents a medical doctor (MD), doctor of osteopathy (DO), nurse practitioner (NP), or physician assistant (PA). Treatment interventions are covered in various sections. However, each member of the healthcare team should only act within his or her scope of practice and follow facility policies and procedures.

The three authors of the first edition brought more than 80 years of combined nursing experience together with their shared common passion for the topic of triage to create a needed resource for healthcare teams. The first edition won third place in the 2015 *American Journal of Nursing* Book of the Year Awards in the critical care/emergency category. The authors reached out to other professionals around the country, who contributed and reviewed chapters, in their quest to bring this book to the highest possible level of functionality for the frontline triage nurse and others practicing triage.

The second edition doubled the number of content reviewers, strengthening the team with leaders from within the Emergency Nurses Association and further expanding to include international reviewers. This team of authors, contributors, and reviewers has nearly 700 years of collective nursing experience. No other source is available on this topic that brings together the expertise of so many valuable professionals. Some readers may want to read this book cover to cover, while others may stick it in their lab coat pocket and pull it out for use as a quick resource to answer a clinical question. Perhaps it will be most helpful to novice readers, who will benefit from the concise expertise contained in this book before "learning it the hard way," one patient at a time.

Contact hours for continuing education credits may be awarded by completing associated post-tests. Access test questions and further instructions via http://connect.springerpub.com/content/book/978-0-8261-4851-3 *or by scanning the QR code with your smartphone.*

Lynn Sayre Visser
Anna Sivo Montejano

~A Heartfelt Thank You~

Valerie Aarne Grossman was the third author for the first edition of *Fast Facts for the Triage Nurse: An Orientation and Care Guide in a Nutshell*. The expertise Valerie brought to the book was pivotal to the overall layout, quality, and award-winning success of the first edition. She selflessly devoted countless hours of time to mentor two new authors eager to make a dream become a reality. Valerie made the difficult decision to step back from the second edition of this book to give her attention to other life commitments.

Valerie,
Your presence during the development of the second edition was surely missed, but we sincerely hope we've made you proud. As Flavia once said, "Some people come into our lives and quickly go. Some stay for a while and leave footprints on our hearts. And we are never ever the same." Thank you for touching the depths of our hearts and for giving us the wings to fly.

Much Love and Gratitude, Lynn and Anna

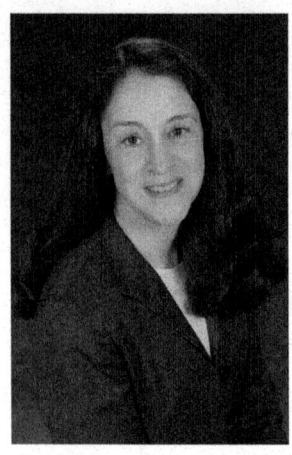

Valerie Aarne Grossman, MALS, BSN, NE-BC, is a registered nurse with over 36 years of heterogeneous nursing experience in direct patient care, hospital leadership, and professional service and as a nurse author. Her areas of practice expertise have included emergency nursing, nursing leadership, telephone triage nursing, and radiology nursing. She has been an active volunteer with nursing organizations, including Emergency Nurses Association, Association for Radiologic and Imaging Nursing, and RAD-AID.org, as well as serving on boards of directors, including the New York State Board for Nursing and the University of Rochester's Research Subjects Review Board, and numerous editorial boards (*American Journal of Interventional Radiology, Journal of Radiology Nursing*, SCOREBoard: Stakeholders for Care in Oncology & Research for the Elderly, and the International Advisory Board for Nurse Education Today). She has authored (or coauthored) numerous peer-reviewed publications, including six book titles (10 editions), six book chapters, and 29 articles. She is the recipient of numerous awards, including the American Nurses Association's Honorary Nursing Practice Award, the Association of Radiologic and Imaging Nursing's Nurse of the Year Award, and Cortland Senior High School's Wall of Fame. Her advocacy for the bedside nurse drives her passion for professional involvement and dedication to creating tools that will be most helpful to them. She believes it is an honor to take care of each patient she encounters during their most vulnerable times in their health crisis or journey.

Acknowledgments

To our superstar editor, Elizabeth Nieginski, and her supportive assistant, Rachel Landes, thank you for your endless positive energy, never-ending encouragement, and for always being quick to reply as questions came up. Grateful for you both for making this project easy and enjoyable to tackle.

To our contributors who have been on this journey with us, we are eternally grateful for each of you. Your knowledge, expertise, and evidence-based research created not only interesting reading but a strong foundation for both those seeking to understand the triage role for the very first time and those who have been in the triage role for years.

To our reviewers, thank you for stepping up to the plate time and time again and for sharing your expertise from all areas of the globe. From the Netherlands to Australia, to the East and West Coasts of the United States, and many areas inbetween, you provided a glimpse into the delivery of emergency care in rural and urban environments as well as on military bases. You all rock!

Many thanks to the Emergency Nurses Association (ENA). Our affiliation with this great organization has opened so many doors for our team and has provided us with unlimited resources, networking opportunities, and professional growth. In fact, our ENA connection is how we met many of the individuals associated with this book. This team of authors, contributors, and reviewers brings a combined total of nearly 700 years of nursing experience, more than 475 years of membership with ENA, almost 400 years as Certified Emergency Nurses, and decades of other experience as Certified Pediatric Emergency Nurses, Certified Flight Registered Nurses, Trauma Certified Registered Nurses, and Certified CriticalCare Nurses. In addition, this team has contributed countless volunteer hours holding board and committee member positions, serving at the local, national, and international level.

Lynn Sayre Visser: To my husband, Scott, and the other rocks in my life, thank you for your endless love and support. To my three teenage boys, Chase, Colton, and Brody, the world is full of opportunities; don't let them pass you by. Always remember there is no such thing as failure; rather learn from each experience, no matter what it looks like, and enjoy the ride! To the many patients, colleagues, and friends I have crossed paths with, I feel so blessed to have had the honor to be there during some of your most intimate and vulnerable moments. Some of you have said I touched your lives and for that I am grateful, but truly I feel most fortunate to have had the depths of my heart touched by you. Lastly, Anna, you are a bright spot in my life day in and day out; never lose your radiance as your steady glow continually sparks my desire to be the best I can be. Thank you for the years of friendship, learning, and laughs.

Anna Sivo Montejano: Thank you again Phil for supporting me with the second edition of *Fast Facts for the Triage Nurse*. I cannot tell you what it means to me to have you by my side every day as I grow professionally in a career I love so much. To my three grown children, Zsuzsa, Michael, and Marcus, don't ever stay stagnant. Seek out your dreams, grab hold of them, and don't let go. Determination, focus, and drive will get you to where you want to be. Never give up and remember, "Stay shredded!"

Finally, to my good friend Lynn, thank you for your friendship and encouragement. We have achieved so many things together that I never dreamed of and it is because of you! You amaze me every day with your ability to persevere when life throws you curve balls. Thank you for your amazing friendship.

Setting the Stage for Success at Triage

1

Orienting to Triage

Lynn Sayre Visser

Embarking on triage orientation is both an exciting and a scary time in a nurse's career due to the geographical isolation of the triage area and the independent decision-making required. Whether you practice in an ED, urgent care center, telephone triage facility, or prehospital setting, new concepts intertwined with potentially different protocols and processes can leave you feeling uneasy. However, with a comprehensive orientation and the right perspective, the rewards that come with working in triage can be greater than the stressors imposed.

Because the triage nurse makes quick decisions that can be the difference between life and death, excellent critical thinking skills and judgment are essential. In addition, the triage nurse must have the ability to multitask while simultaneously considering the needs of patients, colleagues, and the department as a whole. Triage orientation is critical to high-quality patient outcomes and a nurse's success in the triage role.

Upon conclusion of this chapter, you will be able to:

1. Define triage.
2. State the recommended qualifications for a triage nurse.
3. State the purpose of triage orientation.
4. Describe how to prepare for triage orientation.
5. List resources available to enhance the triage education experience.

WHAT IS TRIAGE?

Triage is a dynamic process. The word *triage* is derived from the French verb *trier*, which means "to sort." A person can be triaged anywhere, at any time, with only a moment's notice, and may be triaged in the ambulance bay, in the hospital parking lot, or on the floor of the waiting room. Triage is not isolated to one location but rather it is a *process*; patients are sorted upon arrival and re-sorted frequently throughout their stay.

Many practicing triage nurses find they informally triage patients all day long. This assessment takes place in the grocery store, health club, and while riding the elevator at work. Consider the person you see in the grocery store checkout line, wearing flip-flops. The pitting edema protruding beyond the flip-flop straps is hard to miss. You begin to scan the person from head to toe. You focus on his or her respiratory effort and wonder what the pulse oximetry and heart rate might reveal. This practice of performing spontaneous assessments all day long develops as a habit for nurses and translates to valuable skills that can be utilized in the triage work setting.

The goal of the triage nurse is to determine:

- How sick is the patient?
- How quickly the patient needs to be seen by a medical provider (determined by acuity level)?

Many healthcare facilities have a designated "triage room." This location is merely that—a room in which to store needed supplies that serves as a functional location for triage when the time is appropriate. However, the triage room must *never* be misinterpreted as the only place triage can occur. Triaging patients in the *most* appropriate setting and getting each patient to the *right* treatment location in the time frame necessary to promote best outcomes and reduce mortality is a vital aspect of the triage nurse's role.

RECOMMENDED QUALIFICATIONS OF A TRIAGE NURSE

Before orienting to triage, the orientee and leadership or education team should determine if recommended qualifications to work in triage have been met. According to the Emergency Nurses Association (ENA, 2017), time as an ED nurse is not the determining factor for being qualified for triage; rather, experience in conjunction with formalized triage training, certifications, and specific qualities is suggested.

Qualifications

Recommended qualifications include (but are not limited to):

- Registered nurse or nurse practitioner
- Completion of a formalized triage training program
- Education and documented competency using a valid and reliable triage system
- Completion of a clinical orientation to triage with a dedicated preceptor
- Strong critical-thinking and interviewing skills
- Exceptional interpersonal, communication, and leadership skills
- Solid clinical and physical assessment skills
- Ability to multitask, collaborate, and work under stress
- Ability to educate, delegate, and demonstrate sensitivity to cultural awareness
- Understanding of facility policies and procedures, departmental flow, and treatment areas
- For pediatric and older adult triage, an understanding of developmental stages and physiological differences

According to ENA (2017), a minimum of one year of emergency nursing experience is recommended before taking on the triage role. Additionally, some triage education companies and facilities suggest a minimum of one year's experience at that specific facility before embarking on triage orientation. This time frame gives the nurse ample time to learn facility-specific policies and procedures and so on.

COURSES AND CERTIFICATIONS

Courses and certifications that support the nurse in preparing for the triage role include:

- Certified Emergency Nurse (CEN)
- Certified Pediatric Emergency Nurse (CPEN)
- Trauma Certified Registered Nurse (TCRN)
- Basic Life Support (BLS)
- Basic Disaster Life Support (BDLS)
- Advanced Cardiac Life Support (ACLS)
- Trauma Nursing Core Course (TNCC)
- Advanced Disaster Life Support (ADLS)
- Emergency Nurse Pediatric Course (ENPC)
- Pediatric Advanced Life Support (PALS)
- Geriatric Emergency Nurse Education (GENE)
- Customer service/patient experience training
- Other courses mandated by the organization or governing agencies

> **Fast Facts**
>
> Active membership in at least one professional nursing organization (e.g., Emergency Nurses Association) creates a strong foundation for continued growth within the nursing profession. Networking opportunities, access to nursing forums, and educational offerings will help you develop into the triage nurse you want to be!

PURPOSE OF TRIAGE ORIENTATION

A thorough orientation to triage provides the foundational skills to build upon in the months and years ahead. The orientation should be designed to prepare a person for success and serves many purposes that include:

Understanding the Triage Role

- Gaining confidence in the triage role
- Decreasing stress by developing an understanding of the triage nurse role
- Acquiring tips for enhancing productivity at triage
- Improving job satisfaction

Advancing Current Knowledge

- Developing strong customer service techniques to utilize at triage
- Gaining awareness about compassion fatigue and empathy burnout
- Managing families and their reactions to stress
- Understanding how cultural beliefs and language barriers impact the delivery of care
- Developing competency and improving patient care outcomes
- Learning how to initiate advanced triage protocols

Understanding Triage Flow

- Prioritizing an influx of patients in a short time frame
- Learning when to perform a rapid triage assessment versus a comprehensive triage assessment
- Understanding patient flow, acuity assignment, and priority setting
- Learning how to work with a physician, physician assistant, or nurse practitioner at triage

Identifying "Red Flag" Patient Presentations and Enhancing Documentation Skills

- Gaining awareness of high-acuity presentations and "red flag" findings
- Learning how to best document chief complaints and associated symptoms
- Acquiring tips on working with the electronic medical record (EMR)
- Developing skills to keep patients and staff safe

Understanding Policies and Procedures

- Understanding legal concerns (e.g., provisions of the Emergency Medical Treatment and Active Labor Act [EMTALA] and Health Insurance Portability and Accountability Act [HIPAA] in order to decrease liability)
- Gaining knowledge in the medical screening exam (MSE)
- Understanding facility policies, procedures, and resource availability
  - Availability of a labor and delivery department, cardiac catheterization lab, trauma team, and so on

TRIAGE ORIENTATION

In preparing for triage orientation, the orientee may or may not have an opportunity to choose who shows him or her the ins and outs of triage. Nursing leadership or educators should be actively involved in carefully selecting triage preceptors. The preceptors chosen should be role model staff members who are passionate about teaching and who meet the recommended triage qualifications. From the time we are children, our parents, teachers, coaches, friends, and family share their wisdom, shaping us into the individuals we become. Nursing is the same in that our practice is strongly influenced by other nursing professionals. The right preceptor can make all the difference in a person's orientation and future success at triage.

Fast Facts

- Advanced planning to prepare for triage orientation and ensuring a good preceptor–orientee match is paramount.
- Triage orientation should involve preceptors who will guide, challenge, and support the learning process. Gaining knowledge and exposure to a multitude of experiences during the triage orientation best prepares a person for success at triage.

Selecting the Right Preceptors for Triage Orientation

Triage is an art and science that requires continued growth and development. When contemplating which staff might be best for orienting nurses to triage, consider the following:

- Does the person possess excellent clinical and critical-thinking skills?
- Does the person have sufficient triage experience?
- Is the person enthusiastic and does he or she have the desire to precept with a positive attitude?
- Does the preceptor meet the ENA-recommended triage qualifications?
- Does the person possess effective communication skills?
- Is the person respected by peers for his or her priority-setting abilities at triage?
- Can this person provide constructive criticism?
- Is the person open to receiving constructive criticism from others?
- Is the person knowledgeable about departmental flow?
- Will the person push the orientee to his or her potential?
- Does the person consistently identify unstable patients and assign accurate triage acuity levels?
- Is the person self-motivated to learn and advance his or her precepting and nursing skills?
- Has the person attended preceptor courses and gained knowledge in adult learning principles?
- Will the preceptor maximize the orientation time?

Difficulties can arise between the preceptor and orientee during triage orientation when differences exist, including:

- Expectations
- Values and beliefs
- Personalities
- Past life experiences
- Cultural backgrounds
- Generational differences
- Variation in learning and teaching styles

Efforts to create a positive learning experience for the orientee should be made. Being aware of these differences can help management teams and nurse educators best match the preceptor and orientee.

Communication

Communication *throughout* the triage orientation is essential. Although your organization may have clear objectives for orientation, the orientee should develop personal objectives that are communicated to the preceptor. If the orientee's goals are clearly expressed, the preceptor can best help the orientee achieve them. At times during the orientation, miscommunication may occur. Building the relationship on open and honest communication is imperative. A manager or nurse educator should follow up with the orientee and preceptor to provide support and evaluate if the orientation is meeting the expectations of all involved.

Equipment Lists

Knowing where to find supplies and emergency equipment in the triage area is critical. The unique layout of the triage area often creates systems that may not be uniform with other supplies within the facility. Ensure familiarity with the location of basic equipment, including the following:

- Emergency supplies such as oral airways, bag valve mask, crash cart, and delivery tray
- Code blue button, panic button, emergency numbers
- Stabilization/immobilization devices (e.g., cervical collars, backboards)
- Electrocardiogram machine
- Blood pressure cuffs and pulse oximeters in all sizes
- Blood glucose machines
- Emesis basins, specimen cups, bandaging supplies (e.g., gauze, scissors, saline)
- Personal protective equipment (e.g., gloves, gowns, face shields)
- Downtime slips and paperwork in case of EMR updates or system failures

Teamwork

Although triage may be a geographically isolated area, the role the triage nurse plays is an integral component of the treatment team. Communication with the charge nurse or patient flow coordinator regarding incoming patients and their acuity levels is critical to departmental flow and patient safety. A successful triage orientation requires a team approach to ensure the orientee grasps essential concepts and understands processes unique to the triage area. Acquiring the skills needed to effectively function at triage is beneficial to other staff on the treatment team once the orientee is practicing solo. Thus, throughout this book, content covered will build critical thinking skills and include key concepts to support success at triage.

COMPLETION OF TRIAGE ORIENTATION

Completion of the triage orientation is the first step in beginning a new chapter of nursing experiences. The challenges posed at triage are unlike any others. Often, the triage nurse is the first clinical person who sets the tone for the patient experience and patient outcome. Working with the human dynamics of patients and families in a time of crisis can be overwhelming, but the triage nurse has a unique opportunity to make a difference in the lives of others. Providing each patient presenting to triage with an accurate, unbiased, and nonjudgmental assessment, coupled with caring and compassion, is vital to every patient encounter.

Remember, even though orientation may be complete, the learning should never stop. Even the most seasoned and experienced triage nurses have times of uncertainty in the triage role. No nurse is ever too old, too smart, or too experienced to consult with a fellow nurse or medical provider. A commitment to lifelong learning is vital to your role in nursing and is a critical component to growing into an exceptional triage nurse.

Fast Facts

- Each patient presenting for medical care deserves an unbiased assessment.
- Personal judgments should never influence triage decision-making.
- Although the triage assignment may feel isolating at times, the triage nurse is an integral part of the team.
- Always strive to keep learning so you can continually grow in your clinical knowledge and patient assessment skills. Your commitment to excellence will be a blessing to your patients.

RESOURCES

Although your facility may have a triage orientation program, additional resources to support triage education can be valuable. Appendix A: Resources at the end of this text offers other ideas for enhancing the orientation. These resources include books, formalized live and online triage education programs, and websites.

Reference

Emergency Nurses Association. (2017). *Triage qualifications and competency position statement.* Retrieved from https://www.ena.org/docs/default-source/resource-library/practice-resources/position-statements/triagequalificationscompetency.pdf

2

Precepting at Triage

Lynn Sayre Visser

Precepting an individual at triage is an opportunity to shape that nurse's future practice. When the orientee begins practicing in triage on his or her own, this nurse may make potentially life-saving or life-altering decisions about your family members and friends. Therefore, giving the orientee the experiences and education that you would want every nurse to have at triage is crucial. This chapter covers essential skills required of the preceptor and provides tips for creating a positive experience for the triage orientee.

Upon conclusion of this chapter, you will be able to:

1. Explain adult teaching principles.
2. Understand the impact of generational differences in the workplace.
3. List recommended qualifications for a triage preceptor.
4. Explain benefits of precepting at triage.
5. Describe components of the triage orientation.

ADULT TEACHING AND LEARNING PRINCIPLES

Recognizing that adults do not all acquire new knowledge in a similar manner is fundamental to becoming an excellent preceptor. Individuals come to learning situations with varying past experiences and knowledge upon which to build. Understanding the foundation of work and life experience that the individual possesses is important.

Learning Styles

Learning styles vary among individuals. "Learning style refers to the unique way in which a person perceives, interacts with, and responds to a learning situation" (Billings & Halstead, 2009, p. 23). Some adults may know how they learn best while others may be lacking that insight. As a preceptor, being aware of the unique needs of an individual is vital to laying the groundwork for a caring, mutually respectful relationship. Understanding students personally and professionally, their interests, and how they will best engage in the learning experience helps the preceptor work with each individual.

Adult learning theory supports frequent use of a combination of these learning styles:

- Visual
- Auditory
- Kinesthetic (hands-on application)

Fortunately, triage orientation provides an opportunity to regularly incorporate all three of these learning needs. However, knowledge of the orientee's learning style will help the preceptor seek opportunities to meet the individual's needs. Getting orientees involved in the learning process is critical to their success; thus, the more orientation can be fine-tuned to meet individual needs, the more engaged the person will likely be. Learning style assessments can further aid in discovering how the orientee learns (e.g., the Kolb Learning Style Inventory 4.0).

Important principles of adult learning include:

- Positive reinforcement
- Recognition that adults learn at different speeds

Asking the Right Questions

Asking the orientee to share the learning methods that are most effective for him or her and the expectations the orientee has for the orientation sets the tone for a positive orientee–preceptor relationship. This approach opens the lines of communication between the orientee and preceptor. Questions to ask the orientee *throughout* the orientation include:

- What are your goals for the triage orientation?
- Is auditory or visual learning better for you or do you prefer both?
- Is the hands-on aspect of learning crucial to your success?
- What can I do as a preceptor to ensure I meet your learning needs?
- Do you have any barriers to learning that I should know?
- Do you have previous experience in triage?
- What is a worry you have about working in triage?

- Do you have fears or misconceptions I can try to alleviate?
- What do you like to do in your spare time?

Although inquiring about interests outside the workplace may seem irrelevant, this question opens the door for finding common interests with the orientee and demonstrates your investment in the person as a whole. Outside interests also serve as an outlet for stress release, which is crucial for any individual. Additionally, the preceptor may learn about other relevant life experiences (e.g., work as a paramedic, customer service representative, sales manager) that may influence the individual's performance in the triage role.

Supporting the Orientee

Patience as a preceptor is essential. We all started with limited triage knowledge. Each triage took longer as a new triage nurse. We may have failed to ask the right questions. Maybe a patient was undertriaged or overtriaged or the essential clinical assessment was missed. Gaining knowledge from each experience is part of the learning process. During orientation, providing the orientee with the same level of support you received or wished you had received while orienting to triage will help foster confidence and prepare the new orientee to practice on his or her own. Provide positive reinforcement and constructive feedback when appropriate and maintain an awareness of both verbal and nonverbal communication.

Fast Facts

Let the orientee see your passion for triage and enthusiasm for sharing knowledge with others. Whether working as a preceptor or as a department role model, the knowledge you impart to others will potentially be shared and continue to influence the practice of nurses over time. Teaching and sharing of expertise is one of those gifts that keeps on giving.

THE GENERATIONAL DIVIDE

The profession of nursing is currently influenced by nurses from four generations. Veteran, Baby Boomer, Generation X, and Millennial (also known as Generation Y) nurses work side by side yet reflect different upbringings, belief systems, and values. Generational differences can create challenges in the workplace if these variances are not recognized. Thus, understanding the differences and similarities between the generations and how to instill a cohesive team environment will help preceptors perform. Table 2.1: The Four Generations in Nursing illustrates these important generational variations.

Table 2.1

The Four Generations in Nursing

Generation	Year Born	Colloquial Name	Life Experiences	Characteristics	Approach to New Technology
Veterans	1925–1945	"Silent Generation"	Experienced World War II and the Great Depression in childhood	Hard working Disciplined Dedicated	Slow to learn new technology
Baby Boomers	1946–1964		Came of age during civil rights protests Caring for kids and aging parents	Question authority Risk takers Feel fulfilled through work	Slow to learn new technology
Generation X	1965–1980		Many were raised in single-parent families that were money conscious Exposed to technology in their teen years	Independent Self-reliant Self-motivated Instant gratification Desire mentoring Enjoy work/life balance	Understand technology but are slower to adapt than their Generation Y counterparts
Generation Y	1981–2000	"Net Generation" "Millennials"	Grew up with technology	Multitaskers Desire for constant feedback Enjoy work/life balance	Adapt to new technology easily Expect others to use technology

Increasing utilization of technology in healthcare can certainly create challenges for nurse educators and preceptors. Varying comfort levels with technology and adaptations to technology training sessions will most likely need to be made. For example, if an electronic medical record (EMR) is utilized at your facility, the orientee may require one-on-one interaction or additional time learning the computer system.

RECOMMENDED QUALIFICATIONS FOR A TRIAGE PRECEPTOR

Precepting at triage should be a role that is fulfilled by well-qualified individuals who possess a can-do and will-do attitude. A person's years of experience at triage should not be the deciding factor in determining whether he or she is capable of precepting but rather clinical expertise coupled with enthusiasm and a passion for teaching should be given importance. Knowledge is gained most easily when energy and excitement for the topic is conveyed (Svinicki & McKeachie, 2011). Recommended qualifications for the triage preceptor are discussed in Chapter 1: Orienting to Triage.

Desired Traits in a Triage Preceptor

Additional traits of a triage preceptor include:

- Clinical excellence
- Reliability
- Approachability
- Compassion and empathy
- Enthusiasm
- Familiarity with generational differences
- Strong communication/customer service skills
- Self-motivation

BENEFITS OF PRECEPTING

Staff who precept orientees experience many benefits. Some of the rewards noted may include:

- Personal satisfaction from helping orientees develop professionally
- Opportunity to share knowledge with other nurses
- Growth of self-knowledge derived from the need to understand and explain triage concepts
- Further development of critical thinking skills
- Recognition from peers and managers
- Career advancement
- Giving back to the future of nursing

IDEAS FOR THE ORIENTATION

By the time the orientee is ready for the didactic portion of the triage clinical orientation, hopefully classroom training has been completed and the orientee has a general understanding of triage policies and procedures, a valid and reliable triage acuity scale, and the unique aspects of the triage area. During the orientation process, the preceptor should maximize the time spent with the orientee. Ways to effectively use the orientation time include learning about available resources, policies and procedures, and skills and processes.

Resources

- Have the orientee:
  - Go on a scavenger hunt to find needed triage supplies.
  - Locate electrocardiogram machines and wheelchairs.
  - Learn where supplies needed to stock the triage area are located.
- Discuss with the orientee:
  - The availability of security (e.g., panic buttons, emergency numbers)
  - Use of notification devices (e.g., code blue button, walkie-talkies)
  - Continuing education opportunities and how to access them

Policies and Procedures

- Explain legal concerns at triage, including the Emergency Medical Treatment and Active Labor Act (EMTALA), medical screening exam (MSE), and Health Insurance Portability and Accountability Act (HIPAA).
- Discuss mandated documentation for triage.
- Review requirements for paperwork and the EMR.
- Review policies and procedures of triage acuity levels.
- Evaluate the orientee's understanding of triage acuity levels.
- Review policies for common patient circumstances (e.g., "left without being seen," "against medical advice").
- Review the facility's advanced triage protocols.
- Discuss facility-specific limitations (e.g., no labor and delivery capability, no trauma surgeon availability).
- Review disaster and active shooter/active violence policies and resources.
- Discuss facility lockdown policy and procedures.

Skills and Processes

- Discuss and role model the triage process and patient flow.
- Discuss how to work with other staff at triage (e.g., providers, unlicensed personnel).

- Review the importance of communication and active listening at triage.
- Discuss trauma at triage, team members to activate, whom to call, and patient placement.
- Review "red flag" patient presentations and questions and assessments to consider.
- Discuss and demonstrate the use of customer service skills at triage.
- Demonstrate differences when triaging adult, pediatric, and older adult patients.
- Observe the orientee during triage of adult, pediatric, and older adult patients.
- Review self-care practices (e.g., stress alleviation, avoiding burnout, and compassion fatigue).

Evaluation Techniques

- Discuss the value of self-reflection to enhance the learning experience.
- Discuss the tools utilized to evaluate the orientee.
- Perform chart reviews and evaluate the appropriateness of the triage acuity level assigned.

Additional examples of points to consider during the triage orientation will be threaded throughout future chapters and can help in developing the orientation.

COMPLETION OF TRIAGE ORIENTATION

During the triage orientation, evaluation tools that are evidence-based and supported by facility policies and procedures should be utilized to aid in determining if the orientee is ready for the triage assignment. As a preceptor, your responsibility is to ensure that the orientee is only released to triage solo once facility-specific orientation objectives are met and competency is validated (see Chapter 5). Although formal written tools will likely be utilized in the evaluation process, informal conversations throughout the triage orientation are also important. Consider the tips below for effectively communicating with orientees.

Crucial Conversations

Crucial conversations regarding the orientee's performance can be challenging. However, accurately evaluating the orientee for safe practice at triage is an essential component of precepting. When speaking to an orientee who is having difficulty, use the following guidelines:

- *Provide timely feedback:* Regular, constructive feedback, given both orally and in writing, will minimize surprises at the end of the

orientation. Set orientees up to succeed, and if all else fails, let them know where they stand on a *regular* basis. No one wants to feel they were blindsided at the end of an orientation period, and this practice will alleviate stress for both the preceptor and orientee.
- *Control emotions and avoid defensive behavior:* Mastering this skill can be challenging, especially when experiencing frustration with an orientee. The preceptor needs to think about what to say and how to say it before approaching the orientee. Put yourself in the position of the orientee and think about how the information will be perceived.
- *Address the right problem:* Consider what needs to be tackled so the right results can be achieved.
- *Change the orientee's perspective:* If the orientee's performance raises concerns about patient safety, consider explaining how his or her behavior can potentially impact the patient outcome. The preceptor should think, "What are the consequences of the behavior?" and address the concerns with the orientee.

Giving Praise

Praise is also a critical element of the orientation. Even an orientee who excels will want to know where he or she stands. Some may think no news is good news, but is that enough? Praise serves as both a reward and a motivational tool and should be delivered appropriately to have the greatest impact.

- *Prepare to give praise:* This meaningful moment should receive the same or more preparation as delivering constructive criticism. Make your comments count!
- *Be specific:* Set your standards and expectations early in the orientation and compliment the orientee when expectations are being met. For example, explain that *when* you triaged the patient, *what happened* was you picked up on the subtle symptoms, raising concern of a myocardial infarction, and *the result of your actions* was the identification of a potentially life-threatening condition. When you add that the patient went into cardiac arrest the minute he or she was placed on the gurney, your orientee will feel his or her actions in identifying the sick patient were appropriate!
- *Timely feedback:* Timeliness is essential in providing praise so the orientee remembers the details of the situation. Praise also gives momentum for continuing to perform well and builds confidence.

TIPS FOR NURSING LEADERSHIP AND NURSING EDUCATORS

Ways to support your preceptors include:

- Providing preceptors with training in adult teaching and learning principles, effective communication skills, and conflict management

- Dedicating time to the review of standards of care and policies and procedures
- Selecting preceptors who meet facility or nationally recommended triage qualifications
- Listening to the preceptor if concerns about the orientee arise
- Checking in with the preceptor and orientee throughout the orientation so no surprises develop regarding the orientee's performance
- Considering generational, cultural, and personality differences before matching preceptors and orientees
- Growing a pool of triage preceptors to avoid preceptor burnout
- Providing preceptor training in how best to utilize department resources
- Developing a preceptor committee to enhance communication and ensure the same orientation principles are implemented by all preceptors (e.g., feedback, praise)

Fast Facts

- As a preceptor, commit to being a lifelong learner. To keep up with the ever-changing healthcare system, you must seek learning opportunities and attend continuing education courses.
- Orientees often say knowledge is gained most easily when energy and excitement is relayed by the preceptor. Be a role model!
- Empathize with the orientee. Provide the level of high-quality training that you would want for yourself.

References

Billings, D. M., & Halstead, J. A. (2009). *Teaching in nursing: A guide for faculty* (3rd ed.). St Louis, MO: Elsevier Saunders.

Svinicki, M., & McKeachie, W. J. (2011). *McKeachie's teaching tips: Strategies, research, and theory for college and university teachers* (13th ed.). Belmont, CA: Wadsworth.

3

Tips for Success at Triage

Lynn Sayre Visser and Anna Sivo Montejano

Working in triage can be overwhelming. The fast-paced environment, vast knowledge required, and the unpredictable nature of the triage area can leave even seasoned triage nurses feeling the stress. Emergency nursing leaders were asked to share their techniques for delivering quality care at triage, how they nurture themselves while in the triage role, and how they promote efficient departmental flow, all while keeping patient safety as the primary goal. This chapter includes tips, wisdom, and insights from nurses who have years of experience working in the trenches and their suggestions for setting oneself up for success at triage.

Upon conclusion of this chapter, you will be able to:

1. Identify a minimum of three tips you can incorporate into your triage practice.
2. Reflect on your own triage success tips that you can share with other triage nurses.
3. Identify one method of sharing triage tips that can be incorporated in your facility.

TRIAGE TIPS AND RATIONALE

Erik Angle, RN, MICN, MEP, Roseville, California, California

- Take the initiative to learn ahead of time what role you may hold if a disaster occurs either within or outside your facility. Participate

in training, drills, and exercises so you are prepared in the event disaster strikes.
- As a triage nurse, situational awareness is essential in identifying potential threats of violence. If your instincts sense a threat, act on those senses. Your actions can potentially be the difference in saving lives.
- If multiple patients present with similar signs and symptoms unusual for the season (e.g., flu-like symptoms, febrile illness in midsummer) or from a similar geographical region (e.g., persons attending a same gathering or public special event), consider a potential biological agent exposure.

Shelley Cohen, MSN, RN, CEN, Franklin, Tennessee

- Never make an assumption based on only one sense (what you see, hear, smell, touch). What looks, sounds, smells, and feels normal in and of itself may actually be a "red flag" finding when you engage *all* of your senses.
- Never hesitate to collaborate with a peer or provider on duty when unsure of a triage decision. The triage nurse cannot operate in a vacuum (isolation). Although physically the triage nurse typically works independently of other team members, always reach out for another opinion when needed.
- Learn to document your triage note in a manner that validates your triage decision. The only person who can clinically capture the patient presentation at the time of triage is the triage nurse. When retrospective review is required for legal or other purposes, you want to be sure your words "paint a picture" of this patient's status at the time of triage.

Dawn Friedly Gray, MSN, RN, CEN, CCRN, Paoli, Pennsylvania

- Find a way to show compassion and caring to every patient you triage. Triage is the first and the most important interaction in setting the tone for your patient's visit. Making a connection and attempting to see why a patient is there through his or her eyes builds trust in the patient–nurse relationship.
- Trust your gut. Sometimes there is no specific clinical presentation or answer to a question that can "explain" why you feel someone needs immediate attention. Following your nursing instincts can save a life. Better to follow one's gut than to regret the decision later.
- You can learn something new every time you triage. Be open to learning and take the time to follow up to see if your assessment was appropriate. We should never stop learning and growing as nurses. Taking the time to review and reflect on our clinical decision-making makes us stronger and keeps us attuned to our own "humanness." It helps us avoid judgmental attitudes and promotes ongoing professional development.

- Triage is a constantly changing process, in terms of patients, priorities, assessments, and charting requirements. Don't allow yourself to become comfortable in a set way. Predictability can increase complacency and jeopardize high-quality care.

Valerie Aarne Grossman, MALS, BSN, RN, NE-BC, Rochester, New York

- Never act surprised by anything you hear, see, smell, or touch. By maintaining professionalism at all times, you encourage the patient and his or her family to trust that you are sensitive to their situation, and building a rapport with them will occur more easily.
- Remember that you are always on stage. You may be the first professional whom patients and families see when they enter the hospital, and you may set the tone for their entire stay. If they see that you are a professional and treat all others with respect, they will be more open to answering your questions honestly and facilitating your ability to triage effectively.
- Hear what the patients are saying; they live with their bodies and their lives more than you do. Not everything we hear in triage makes sense to us. However, don't assume that you are smarter than the patient when it comes to his or her body or life. If the patient says something that doesn't make sense, ask a few more questions instead of being quick to pass judgment on him or her.

Reneé Semonin Holleran, FNP-BC, PhD, CEN, CCRN (emeritus), CFRN and CTRN (retired), FAEN, former editor in chief, Journal of Emergency Nursing *(2006–2013), Salt Lake City, Utah*

- Listen to what patients tell you about their problems. Take a brief history to go along with the chief complaint. PQRST is a great tool for this. Most of the time the patient will tell you what is wrong. The physical assessment or other tests only confirm it.
- Today patients are on a plethora of medications prescribed by multiple providers. These medications are mixed in with over-the-counter medications that cause serious and often chronic side effects that frequently are worked up over and over again. Medications and medication interactions cause many problems that are often mistaken for something else.
- Caring and compassion can go a long way in getting you through a long shift. It takes more effort to be rude than to be kind.

Deb Jeffries, MSN-Ed, RN, CEN, CPEN, Phoenix, Arizona

- Keep an open mind; the "been there, done that; I've seen this a million times before" attitude will end up burning you. It is inherent in what nurses do that we categorize patients by the chief complaint, symptom clusters, and the appropriate corresponding objective assessment. However, we must always be on guard to avoid categorizing and prioritizing patients based on invalid factors such as "drug seekers," "people who are overreacting," and "attention seekers."

- Delete the word *just* from your vocabulary and your thinking when you are at triage. If I could influence one last thing in my career, it would be to eradicate the word *just* from the mindset of every triage nurse worldwide. The word *just* influences, albeit subtly sometimes, how we look at, assess, and determine prioritization of care for the patient. Phrases like *He's just drunk* and *He's just a drug seeker* will affect how we think about the patient. At triage, there is *no one* who is "just" anything.
- Use a systematic approach to everything you do at triage. Using a consistent, systematic approach will help ensure that you do not miss anything. Whether it is how you obtain subjective and objective assessments or how you facilitate reassessments on patients awaiting treatment area placement, a systematic approach will help you go home at the end of your shift knowing that you have provided the best care possible to all those you have triaged.
- Although at triage we are more often than not overwhelmed and pressured to get patients seen quickly while making safe decisions regarding prioritization, interventions, and dispositions, making eye contact and smiling warmly at patients and their families is never a waste of time. A "small" gesture such as this can change the entire tone of the visit and help alleviate some of the fear associated with a trip to the ED.

Rebecca S. McNair, RN, CEN, Fairview, North Carolina

- Obtain as much clinical education as possible, including advanced cardiac life-support training, trauma nursing core course, emergency nurse pediatric course, and especially your certified emergency nurse (CEN) certification. The more clinical knowledge you have, the better prepared you will be to accurately and confidently triage any presentation.
- Engage in professional organizations for professional nursing development. Triage and any point-of-entry process require a holistic and well-developed framework to be highly successful.
- Complete a formal, standardized triage course. A conceptual grasp of the knowledge and skills necessary ensures accurate assignment and disposition of triage acuity level.

Anna Sivo Montejano, DNP, RN, PHN, CEN, Oceanside, California

- Whenever a patient is placed in the triage room, make sure the patient enters first and then the nurse follows. If the nurse needs to exit quickly, due to a dangerous situation, it is easier to do so without the patient blocking the exit. Consider this when escorting a patient to an ED or urgent care bed. Always think

"Safety first." Some patients may be unpredictable, leaving you trapped in the room with no way out!
- No matter what a patient tells you, never appear shocked. This may make the patient feel very uncomfortable. Have the attitude, "I see or hear this all the time!" It can be difficult for a patient to seek help, especially in an embarrassing situation.
- Always put on your "happy face" when greeting your triage patients. Patients may be going through a very stressful situation. They need someone who is compassionate and caring, not a cranky, irritable nurse who presents himself or herself as rude and unkind.
- Overexaggerate when asking patients if they drink alcohol. It's easier for a patient to admit to drinking less than more. Asking whether a patient normally drinks 2 L of whisky a day leaves the patient feeling better, as he or she can reply, "Oh no, just one liter." He or she will also be more honest.
- When evaluating the use of drugs, maintain a matter-of-fact expression, as if you were questioning a person about shortness of breath or chest pain. It is easier for the patient to answer without the addition of a nonverbal stigma being applied. Expressing to the patient, both verbally and nonverbally, that this is "simply a fact" may make it easier for a patient to admit to a drug history.

Lynn Sayre Visser, MSN, RN, PHN, CEN, CPEN, Loomis, California

- Triage is too complex to take the "see one, do one, teach one" approach to orientation. Attending a formalized triage education course should be the foundation of a person's triage orientation and can benefit seasoned triage nurses, too! Once the principles of triage are understood, the appropriate application of concepts in the clinical setting can best be achieved.
- When "the bus lets off" and the waiting room is packed wall to wall, often the tension builds among the triage team. When every second counts more than ever, one must never forget to see each arriving patient as an individual. A compassionate touch of a hand, a warm smile, or a genuine look of concern can go miles toward earning the respect of those waiting. Building rapport with the waiting room crowd is essential to survival at triage! When you set the right tone with each person upon arrival, those in the waiting room will "have your back" if a belligerent patient or irate person steps your way.
- Some of the most treasured gifts I have received in my career have come from my work at triage. No words can adequately represent the personal satisfaction that comes with *recognizing* the person with an atypical myocardial infarction, the letus in danger, or the subtle clues of intimate partner violence and then *acting* on the

best interest of the patient. Cherishing the moments where you make a difference in the patient's outcome will help carry you through the tougher triage shifts.
- Invest in good quality shoes. Find a triage mentor. Share cases. Reflect on your triage shifts. Learn from mistakes. Never think you are too seasoned to mess up. We all have times when we fall flat on our faces. It's the journey—both triumphs and failures—that ultimately make us the best triage nurses we can be.

Polly Gerber Zimmermann, MS, MBA, RN-BC, CEN, FAEN, Indianapolis, Indiana

- When building rapport with the pediatric patient, you can't go wrong overestimating a young child's age. "Are you seven? Oh, only five. Well, you seem like such a big boy!" You also can't go wrong telling parents what a cute and nice baby they have. What to do if the baby is not "pretty"? Say "That is *some* baby" or compliment the cute outfit. Now you've started on the right foot, by showing how perceptive and smart you are as a nurse!
- Insist on a lunch break. I routinely worked 12-hour shifts without any break when things were hectic, to avoid the perception that the triage nurse was "sitting" while the rest of staff were "running around." Keep drinking water throughout the shift regardless. One of the first signs of dehydration is fatigue. Everyone needs a break. Even 5 minutes away will make you more effective.
- Toward the end of the triage interaction, use a scripted phrase to show you care. My favorite comments are "That looks sore"; "I'm sorry this happened to you. I'm sure you didn't plan to be here"; and "We'll take good care of you." This approach works to reassure the patient and show your empathy without trying to be original and creative when you are busy.
- Overestimate the time for anything (obtaining a bed, seeing the physician, going to radiology, etc.). Patients respond more positively when something happens before they expect it. No one likes to be the bearer of unpleasant news, so the temptation is strong to underestimate the time it will take for actions to occur. In the end, though, this just irritates patients more.
- The seriously ill are sometimes too sick to speak up. Therefore, do what you are supposed to do, whether you think it is needed or not. By checking all newly arrived patients, I found a patient who had been transported by ambulance with "hysterical back pain" who had rapidly progressing Guillain–Barré syndrome. By always doing an across-the-room assessment, I discovered a dusky infant with bradycardia and an asthmatic patient just before respiratory arrest occurred. The consistent theme was that none of them were asking for help.

> **Fast Facts**
>
> Ensure the triage nurse receives regular breaks. When a person feels run down, critical thinking skills may be impaired and compassion and caring can be difficult to deliver. Breaks recharge an individual so high-quality patient care can be provided.

REFLECTION

Reflection is an essential component of professional growth. Learning from past experiences provides opportunity to incorporate knowledge gained into future practice. This chapter encompasses triage tips from nurses who have worked in the trenches and have learned through their experiences how to succeed during a shift in triage.

What triage tips do you have that you can bestow on others? We challenge you to reflect on your own practice and share triage tips with coworkers at your facility.

- Develop a bulletin board where staff can post their ideas.
- Share a tip of the day at change of shift.
- Create a Triage Tip Binder or "Triage Tip Electronic Folder" with subcategories (e.g., security issues), which all triage staff can access in the triage area.

As we each reflect on what has and has not worked for us at triage, we can create a better, safer, higher-quality triage area and change the face of triage, one tip at a time!

> **Fast Facts**
>
> - Compassion and caring should be hallmarks of the care you deliver.
> - Ongoing reflection is the key to fine-tuning your triage practice.
> - If a patient presentation seems perplexing, consult with a colleague or medical provider. You should never feel alone at triage, but rather you should seek the help you need to act in the best interest of the patient *always*.

4

Personal Awareness for the Triage Nurse

Anna Sivo Montejano

Working in a stressful environment like triage can take a toll on a person. Self-awareness of one's emotions, feelings, and behavior is vital if the triage nurse is to function effectively. Irrespective of whether a nurse works in an urgent care center, in an ED, or as a telephone triage nurse, stressors impact individuals differently. The effects of these stressors can appear insignificant initially, but the overwhelming emotions the nurse experiences daily can lead to physical or psychological crisis. This chapter provides information for handling self-awareness stressors that can affect the nurse's ability to work in a demanding environment. Being aware of these factors can assist the nurse in keeping balance in his or her life.

Upon conclusion of this chapter, you will be able to:

1. Define compassion fatigue.
2. Describe examples of how lateral violence affects patients.
3. Explain empathy burnout.

COMPASSION FATIGUE

Healthcare providers are confronted daily with emotionally challenging situations, which can tear at one's inner soul. We hear stories of pain, loss, and fear while often simultaneously seeing the tears of our patients and their families. Containing our own emotions can be difficult at times. How do healthcare providers suppress the anguish that is a part of their daily routine? Recognizing that healthcare providers are at risk for compassion fatigue is important.

Compassion fatigue results from caring for individuals with physical and emotional suffering, which diminishes the care providers' emotional, physical, and spiritual well-being.

Populations Vulnerable to Compassion Fatigue

- ED personnel
- Intensive care personnel
- First responders
- Firefighters
- Police officers
- Chaplains

Signs and Symptoms of Compassion Fatigue

- Easily frustrated or irritated
- Physical, emotional, and mental exhaustion
- Difficulty getting to work
- Diminished interaction with others
- Losing compassion
- Feeling tired even after a good night's sleep

Prevention of Compassion Fatigue

Understanding the intricacies of compassion fatigue can help healthcare providers cope with their emotions rather than concealing them. A path of self-destruction can develop if the symptoms are not addressed appropriately. The treatment for compassion fatigue includes:

- Exercise
- Articulating your needs
- Adequate sleep
- Self-care
- Seeking support from others
- Validating your feelings with others who can relate
- Obtaining medical help if needed, but *do not self-medicate*

Fast Facts

- Awareness of physical and emotional pain experienced can lead to identifying compassion fatigue, which can help one seek appropriate intervention and a return to a healthy lifestyle.

LATERAL VIOLENCE

Lateral violence, also termed *horizontal violence*, is bullying in the workplace. Lateral violence can cause stress and intimidation toward the victim. If experienced on a continuous basis, lateral violence may cause individuals to leave the profession of nursing.

Three Forms of Lateral Violence

- Physical
  - Inappropriate sexual innuendoes and touching (e.g., unwanted back rubbing)
- Verbal
  - Condescending and/or rude comments
  - Verbal attacks
- Psychological
  - Attacks on one's integrity
  - Refusing to offer assistance
  - Eye rolling
  - Not working as a team
  - Gossiping about the individual
  - Judged constantly by others

You may have experienced one or more forms of lateral violence at some point in your career. Perhaps you assigned a high acuity level to a patient and were met with derogatory comments from coworkers. As professionals, we must remember that often the entire picture is not visible to the eye. For example, consider a patient who arrives with minimal swelling to the forearm, following an insect bite. One nurse may be quick to judge that this should be a low acuity patient. But when the patient's high blood pressure and additional symptoms—including a headache—are considered, the need for a higher acuity level becomes apparent. Comments from other staff regarding triage decision-making should be withheld unless a patient is endangered or feedback is constructive.

Possible Consequences of Lateral Violence

- Errors (e.g., medication, lack of interventions)
- High rate of absenteeism
- Increased staff turnover
- Decreased job satisfaction
- Inadequate communication with the staff member due to intimidation may result in a poor patient outcome

Prevention of Lateral Violence

- Provide education.
- Ensure professional accountability.

- Empower staff to confront issues and promote team building.
- Provide management support.

> **Fast Facts**
>
> Lateral violence leads to significant financial loss each year from absenteeism, lack of work performance, and increased turnover.

EMPATHY BURNOUT

Empathy is an emotional connection with a patient. Empathy burnout is the lack of empathy; the ability to feel connected emotionally is no longer there. This type of burnout can impact patient safety.

Impact of Empathy Burnout on Patient Safety

- Stereotyping individuals and then ignoring what they have to say or are feeling
  - Assuming an individual of a certain ethnicity has no pain because of his or her stoic response
  - Concluding that a crying teenager with complaints of abdominal pain is being overly dramatic because of a recent breakup with his or her significant other
- Assigning a lower acuity level because of personal bias, resulting in an inappropriate disposition

Prevention of Empathy Burnout

- Be aware of your personal bias.
- Take breaks from triage to rejuvenate yourself.
- Work short shifts in triage and rotate to other areas of the department.
- Take time off throughout the year so you can reenergize and best care for others.

> **Fast Facts**
>
> Burnout is another term used to describe continued interpersonal and job-related emotional stressors that can influence the overall effectiveness of an organization.

5

Triage Competency

Shelley Cohen

In the emergency care environment, nurses complete baseline and ongoing education as well as assessment of knowledge and skill in many areas. Examples of these include Advanced Cardiac Life Support (ACLS), use of the fingerstick glucose monitor, and Trauma Nursing Core Course (TNCC). The role of the triage nurse has not historically fit into this list of ongoing education and competency validation, yet triage is the most commonly performed nursing function. This chapter provides a foundation of knowledge to help guide you in the development of triage competency processes while understanding how to differentiate education from competency.

Upon conclusion of this chapter, you will be able to:

1. Differentiate the terms *education* and *competency*.
2. Identify three methods used to validate triage competency.
3. List three essential elements for successful triage competency processes.

EDUCATION VERSUS COMPETENCY

A strong foundation of triage knowledge is imperative in order for the nurse to have successful application in making triage decisions. When the Emergency Nurses Association (ENA) updated their position statement *Triage Qualifications and Competency*, they recognized the "extensive internal base of knowledge" necessary in the triage decision-making process. They also noted the need for triage competency validation to be an ongoing process, not a once-a-year event. Filling the triage knowledge gap occurs by providing the educational component, while demonstrating the ability to apply this knowledge in the actual triage setting is the competency component. Distinguishing your triage education from validating triage competency is essential for attaining consistency in holding staff accountable and ensuring safe triage practices.

Definitions

Education: Providing knowledge that when completed successfully implies the learner has an understanding and awareness of this information

Competency: A display of the ability to apply knowledge/education, skill, and aptitude

At times, both become intertwined as in a course for certification in which the learner is provided with both knowledge and facts as well as a practical application component.

METHODS OF EVALUATING TRIAGE COMPETENCY

A variety of methods exist to demonstrate competency for any nursing skill or knowledge application. Because verification methods do vary, selecting triage competencies that not only reflect critical thinking but also connect to improving triage decisions and patient outcomes is important. The details and elements of triage competency can be integrated directly into the nurse's job description. This brings clarity to the expectations for the triage nurse.

Observation

Develop a list of specific criteria for preceptors to use as a guide when observing new staff in triage. These items may include:

- Customer service perceptions such as how the triage nurse greets the patient and caregiver
- Making eye contact with the patient
- Offering empathy
- Utilizing the correct blood pressure cuff

A sample Triage Competency Validation form is available in Appendix B.

Retrospective Chart Review (Self-Review and/or Peer Review)

Identify the following:

- Frequency of review
- Number of records to review

- Specific documentation elements
- Does the documentation validate the triage level assigned?
- Does the assigned triage level match the practice standard for the facility-designated sorting tool used (e.g., Emergency Severity Index [ESI], Canadian Triage and Acuity Scale [CTAS], Australasian Triage Scale [ATS], Manchester Triage System [MTS])?

Case Scenario/Case Study Packets

Use scenarios that demonstrate the ability to apply critical thinking.

Feedback

Develop a process for staff (including providers) to share their observations of the nurse's ability to consistently apply organizational triage policies and processes, which may include:

- *Posttests*
  - These may be presented in a written format or as a group process to be done orally at the end of a class.
  - The posttest is typically a multiple-choice format that relates directly to the triage course content taught in class or during an online teaching format.
  - Content of the posttest may focus on the triage scoring system used (e.g., ESI, CTAS, ATS, MTS) or it may be extensive and include critical thinking "red flag" cases.

- *Exemplars*
  - Staff submit in writing or as a presentation an actual patient triage that describes the decisions they made and the critical thinking involved in the decision-making. The presentation may occur during a staff meeting, as part of a newsletter, or in an annual competency packet.

COMPONENTS OF TRIAGE COMPETENCY

The three components of competency that should be validated include:

- Critical thinking
- Technical skills
- Interpersonal skills

These three components can be assessed by the following:

- Critical thinking: case scenarios, retrospective chart review
- Technical skills: observation, retrospective chart review
- Interpersonal skills: observation, preceptor feedback, patient complaints/compliments

Use more than one method to verify triage competency to ensure all three components are validated. Engage staff in the development of both triage education and triage competency content. All levels of leadership and educators need to support staff in meeting competency requirements. Provide opportunities and time for retrospective chart reviews as well as schedule time-off or replacement resources so those who need to participate in education and/or remediation efforts can do so. Nurse assignments must reflect those deemed qualified and competent to triage.

Appendix C, Sample Triage Education and Competency Plan, is a form that can be utilized during the triage orientation. For the new graduate nurse, you want to ensure the successful completion of the probationary period prior to participating in triage education. In addition, determine how many direct observation shifts will be required with a preceptor when they begin at triage and then reevaluate the needs of the orientee throughout the orientation.

Fast Facts

Assessing triage competency is far more than determining if the correct sense of urgency was determined. In order to optimize expanding and enhancing the knowledge of the triage nurse, the facility should:

- Develop a written triage competency plan for all skill levels.
- Clarify both education and competency expectations.
- Offer remediation opportunities that promote confidence in triage decision-making.
- Review the triage competency plan annually to ensure the elements remain timely and meet current practice standards.

RETROSPECTIVE CHART REVIEW

Retrospective triage chart reviews are essential components in education and competency and serve different purposes. These reviews can be self-review and/or performed by a peer or nurse educator. See Appendix D for a sample triage retrospective chart review audit form.

Chart Audits for Self-Review

For triage competency self-review, the nurses are provided with a detailed retrospective audit form and then directed as to what charts to pull from patients they triaged. For example, they may be asked to review five adult chest pain and five pediatric abdominal pain presentations. During the self-review process, the triage nurses should be able to identify "red flags" that directed their triage decision as well as any documentation that was possibly lacking. The key question for the nurse to consider is as follows: "Looking back at your triage note now, do you have adequate documentation that supports the triage level selected?"

Chart Audits by Others

The role of the peer or nurse educator reviewer is to provide another set of eyes that can review the chart for specific triage elements and help reinforce the good triage decision-making the nurse has demonstrated. On the other hand, the peer or nurse educator reviewer may identify areas in need of remediation (e.g., documentation, critical thinking, "red flag" observations).

Fast Facts

If retrospective chart reviews are only completed by others, the triage nurse misses the opportunity to self-reflect on his or her triage decision-making. Self-reflection is an essential component of learning and growing as a triage nurse. Therefore, retrospective chart audits completed by both the triage nurse and another source (e.g., peer, educator) provide the optimal opportunity to learn from less-than-ideal decision-making and documentation and to reinforce good decision-making.

II

Point-of-Entry Processes in Triage Nursing

6

The Patient Arrival

Anna Sivo Montejano

When multiple patients present seeking medical care, the triage nurse determines who has the highest priority. This task can be challenging because of the unpredictable influx of patients at different times of the day. The ability to rapidly assess, determine an initial acuity level, and appropriately place patients within the department is imperative to the successful delivery of care. Along with the rapid triage assessment, knowing when to perform a comprehensive triage assessment and the use of critical thinking skills play a critical role in patient care. This chapter discusses the essential information required by the nurse upon the patient's arrival.

Upon conclusion of this chapter, you will be able to:

1. Define the roles of a triage nurse.
2. Explain the purpose of a rapid triage assessment.
3. Summarize the data obtained by a comprehensive triage assessment.

ROLES OF A TRIAGE NURSE

A triage nurse's primary role is to identify the sickest patient so treatment may be rendered without delay. Although it seems that this would be the only function, triage nurses wear many hats to fulfill their job on a daily basis. The following examples are additional roles of the triage nurse:

- *Greeter:* Greets patients on arrival and establishes a warm friendly environment
- *Resource person:* Problem solver (e.g., wheelchair/cervical spine needs)
- *Department expeditor:* Coordinates placement of patients based on department resources
- *Information center:* Provides information and directions to areas in and around the facility (e.g., radiology, labor and delivery, closest pharmacy, and bus stop location)
- *Crowd control:* Keeps track of those who are patients versus family and friends
- *Crisis manager:* Handles distraught family member(s), lost belongings, and so on
- *Safety and security:* Handles the initial contact when an agitated patient needs to be reassured
- *Infection control:* Educates patients about steps that decrease the spread of germs
- *Communicator:* Explains department processes; updates patients, family, and visitors
- *Educator:* Educates about first aid, safety issues (helmets), and healthy living
- *Privacy provider:* Provides a private area when needed for stressful situations
- *Reassessment nurse:* Reevaluates patients who are waiting for treatment

RAPID TRIAGE ASSESSMENT

A rapid triage assessment begins with an across-the-room survey. Visualizing the patient's appearance as he or she enters the facility is the beginning of the rapid triage assessment. A great deal of information can be gathered by visualizing the patient as he or she steps into the waiting room (WR):

- Does the person use a device to assist with ambulation (e.g., cane, walker)?
- Does the facial expression or body language indicate pain?
- What is the skin tone and color?
- Is the gait slow, rapid, absent, or demonstrating signs of weakness?
- Is he or she unresponsive or altered?
- Is there limited eye contact?

- Does the person express fear, anxiety, or agitation?
- Do the clothes give clues to his or her profession (e.g., paint on clothing)?

Gathering information on *every* patient who enters the ED is important to assess for a potential or actual life-threatening condition and enable care to be rendered if needed. A few examples of objective information obtained during the rapid triage assessment include:

- *Airway:* Patent or impaired (e.g., stridor, hoarseness, drooling, facial, or oropharyngeal edema)
- *Breathing:* Unlabored or labored (e.g., accessory muscle use, retractions, nasal flaring)
- *Circulation:* Skin color (e.g., pallor, cyanosis) and moisture (e.g., dry, moist, diaphoretic); pulse rate (e.g., fast or slow) and rhythm (e.g., regular or irregular); obvious bleeding
- *Disability (neurological status):* Level of consciousness including Glasgow Coma Scale (GCS) or alert, verbal, pain, unresponsive (AVPU) scale; muscle strength in upper extremities (e.g., pronator drift, grips) and lower extremities (e.g., ability to lift both legs?)
- *Exposure/environment:* Hyperthermic, hypothermic, or normothermic; presence of objects or forensic evidence requiring preservation

The importance of performing a rapid triage assessment cannot be overemphasized. Imagine a scenario in which 10 patients arrive simultaneously to the ED. If the triage nurse initially performs a lengthy assessment on each individual, the last patient in line may be the sickest. By rapidly assessing each patient for no more than 60 to 90 seconds, the nurse can *best prioritize* patients, ensuring that higher acuity level patients are seen first.

Delay in Care

If a rapid triage assessment is not performed as stated previously, delay in recognizing the patient's severity of illness may result in failure to achieve necessary treatment goals or patient deterioration. The following are examples of situations in which recognition of a high-acuity patient may go unnoticed:

- Dismissing the across-the-room assessment
- Taking care of patients on a first-come, first-served basis
- Triaging all patients quickly but *maintaining* their original order of arrival when additional information is needed (e.g., comprehensive triage assessment)
- Allowing bias to hinder the assessment

> - *Every* patient should have a rapid triage assessment upon arrival.
> - The rapid triage assessment should be completed by a seasoned nurse. There is so much more to triage than solely obtaining the chief complaint.
> - Your senses during the rapid triage assessment may give you a clue as to what is going on with the patient (e.g., fruity acetone breath could indicate elevated blood glucose). Pay attention to your senses and what they may be telling you.

IMMEDIATE BEDDING

Immediate bedding is just what it states: providing a bed for a patient immediately upon arrival to the facility as long as specific criteria are first met. In the past, triage was performed as a step-by-step process that required all steps to occur in a specific sequence for the patient to be seen by a provider. When the patient arrived at the facility, nonmedically trained personnel obtained a chief complaint followed by patient demographic information.

Today, to improve efficiency, safety, and the patient experience, a parallel process is recommended. A triage nurse should be the first person a patient sees upon arrival at the facility. This nurse has the training, along with the assessment and critical thinking skills, to determine the patient's immediate needs. While the rapid triage assessment is being performed and the chief complaint obtained, registration staff can simultaneously gather the minimal data needed to enter the patient into the system. During this initial encounter, the nurse must assess three criteria to determine the need for immediate bedding; *all three must exist* (Triage First Inc., 2018):

- Obviously ill or injured (*or nurse is able to quickly and confidently determine accurate acuity and appropriate disposition*)
- Open bed (*available or able to obtain*)
- Available care provider(s) (*consider the acuity of the patient load*)

Immediate bedding prevents patients from being pulled back and forth from the WR to registration, to the WR, to the triage nurse, and so on, getting them where they need to be—a treatment bed—so care can be initiated. However, an available care provider (e.g., registered nurse, charge nurse) to accept the patient upon placement in the bed is a critical part of the process.

Points to Consider When Practicing Immediate Bedding

- After a rapid triage assessment has been completed, follow the immediate bedding criteria.

- If your facility has an unlicensed assistive staff member (e.g., patient care technician, nurse's aide, emergency room technician), this person would be the ideal choice to escort the patient to a room so the triage nurse can continue triaging. The primary bedside nurse, patient flow coordinator, or charge nurse may also be utilized as a resource for rooming the patient.
    - The triage nurse should *remain at triage* to identify incoming patients and ensure the safety of patients waiting.
- Ensure proper handoff of the new arrival from the triage nurse to the bedside nurse.
- Once handoff has occurred, the bedside nurse will take over care of the patient.
- When selecting the most appropriate room assignment, consider the acuity level of the bedside nurse's current patients. A high-acuity assignment will not allow the bedside nurse to effectively care for the new patient arrival.

If bed availability increases at a time when an influx of lower acuity patients enter the department, the triage nurse may consider placing a patient in a bed even though he or she does not meet the first immediate bedding criteria, "obviously injured or sick." However, it is important to avoid unnecessarily overwhelming the main ED beds, thus ensuring availability for higher acuity patients who may arrive.

Fast Facts

- A rapid triage assessment is performed to identify high-acuity patients and initiate immediate bedding criteria when indicated.
- A patient may arrive with airway, breathing, circulation, and neurological status intact, but some aspect of their presentation (e.g., white particles on clothing) may give you a clue to an exposure that requires immediate isolation to protect other patients, visitors, and staff.
- If a patient states that he or she was involved in a bus accident, explosion, or similar incident, be prepared to initiate a facility disaster response; other patients may be arriving soon. Follow your protocol!

COMPREHENSIVE TRIAGE ASSESSMENT

The comprehensive triage assessment follows the rapid triage assessment and supplies the remainder of the patient's history so that a final triage acuity level can be determined. *On average*, a comprehensive triage should take 2 to 5 minutes; however, there may be times when this process takes longer.

Reasons for a Longer Comprehensive Triage Assessment

- Older adult patient (e.g., delay in motor movement, responds slowly to questions, hard of hearing)
- Patient with numerous medication bottles
- Language barrier
- Patient with multiple layers of clothing
- Patient safety issue (e.g., behavioral health)
- Child who requires an antipyretic
- Confused or uncooperative patient

Not all patients will receive a comprehensive triage assessment upon arrival. When a bed is available and immediate bedding criteria are met, the comprehensive triage will occur at the bedside. With the patient in the room, the physician and nurse can simultaneously hear the history and partake in the physical assessment. This process is efficient and decreases the questioning that the patient experiences.

Information Obtained During the Comprehensive Triage Assessment

- Vital signs
- Weight and height
- Medications
- Complete history (e.g., medical, surgical)
- Allergies to medications and foods
- Screening questions (e.g., intimate partner violence, fall risk)

When obtaining the comprehensive triage assessment, completing the history while simultaneously obtaining the vital signs can save time. Asking for the medication list can help the nurse with information regarding the medical history. For example, when patients are asked about their medical history, they may state only that they have diabetes. However, when specifically asked about medications, a patient may provide information about three medications he or she is taking: an antihypertensive, a lipid-lowering agent, and an oral hypoglycemic. Upon further questioning, the patient may confirm, "Oh yes, I do have high cholesterol and high blood pressure." When the patient is questioned about medications *before* the medical history, this delay in information can be prevented.

Fast Facts

- In some facilities two or more nurses work in the triage area. One nurse should focus on the rapid triage assessment while another nurse should complete the comprehensive triage assessment. Stress the importance of there being one rapid triage assessment nurse who knows all the patients.

(continued)

(*continued*)

- During busy hours, if the rapid triage assessment nurse has no incoming patients to assess, he or she may assist the comprehensive nurse.
- If comprehensive assessments are consistently taking a long time, there may be a breakdown in the process or resources (e.g., lack of support, supplies) or both.
- In facilities where there is only one triage nurse, this nurse will perform a rapid triage assessment on all arriving patients, and when indicated and as time allows, complete a comprehensive triage assessment. If you are performing a comprehensive triage assessment and additional patients arrive:
  - Stop the triage, kindly excusing yourself.
  - Rapidly assess the incoming patient(s).
  - Return to complete the comprehensive triage assessment.

CRITICAL THINKING SKILLS

Critical thinking is used every minute in triage as the nurse assesses patients upon their arrival. As nurses, we use our senses of sight, smell, hearing, and touch while asking questions to gather information. Once the information is gathered, we then critically think, synthesizing the information obtained to determine an accurate acuity level.

Examples of Critical Thinking

- Are the patient's history and medications contributing to the signs and symptoms he or she is exhibiting?
- Is there information that the patient may not be sharing that requires further probing?
- Are illegal substances causing or escalating the signs and symptoms of the patient's complaint?
- Does the information the patient is telling you make sense?
- Has someone accompanied the patient, and is that person having an impact on how much the patient is telling you?
  - For example, a 15-year-old who is complaining of abdominal pain may not disclose that she is pregnant because her mother is sitting next to her.

Intuition is based less on evidence-based practice than on the experiences of the nurse. Some of the phrases used to describe this instinctive feeling are *a gut feeling*, *instinct*, and *a sixth sense*. A seasoned nurse may find it difficult to explain these responses to a novice nurse because they operate outside conscious reasoning. Novice nurses want to know, "How did you know?" when all the nurse can answer is, "I just had a feeling." This ability comes from knowledge and experience.

Examples of a Nurse's Intuition

- The nurse moves a patient with a simple bee sting to a room in front of the nurse's station to be monitored.
    - Twenty minutes later the patient has a cardiac arrest.
- An unkempt female patient arrives via ambulance with abdominal pain and diarrhea. Medics and staff downplay the scenario.
    - One hour later the nurse has an uneasy feeling, looks under the patient's sheet, and visualizes a newborn baby.
- A behavioral health patient has been experiencing seizures while awake. Medical staff attribute the seizures to her behavioral health history, and no CT scan is ordered.
    - The nurse assesses several neurological deficits and advocates for ordering a CT scan of the brain. The patient's diagnosis after the CT scan: malignant brain tumor.

Fast Facts

Intuition can save someone's life. Making a decision without relying on intuition can result in a poor outcome.

Reference

Triage First, Inc. (2018). *ED Triage: Comprehensive Course*. Asheville, NC: Author.

7

The Patient Experience in Triage Nursing

Lynn Sayre Visser

> *In healthcare today, patient satisfaction is more important than ever. Patient satisfaction is linked not only to high-quality clinical care but also to the patient experience. The success of an organization depends on its customers; thus, staff should recognize that both real and perceived experiences impact a person's impression of the service rendered. Because you never get a second chance to make a first impression, making that first interaction a positive experience is essential. Staff training in the delivery of top-notch service is a key element to creating a customer-friendly environment that promotes patient satisfaction. However, no amount of training will enhance the delivery of service for disgruntled staff. Thus, first and foremost, staff must be cared for. Happy staff = happy patients!*

Upon conclusion of this chapter, you will be able to:

1. State two key elements of providing an effective customer experience.
2. List two examples of the right words at the right time.
3. Explain the importance of rounding and reassessments in the waiting room (WR).

PROVIDING A POSITIVE PATIENT EXPERIENCE

Care for Staff First

Providing a positive patient experience does not come easily to all staff, especially unhappy staff. Staff members must first feel *valued* and *cared for* before being asked to deliver excellent service. Staff who are satisfied with their work environment can more easily convey a sense of caring in a genuine tone of voice and with corresponding body language. Thus, measures should be taken to build staff camaraderie and address workplace issues. Consider whether the following issues exist:

- The presence of lateral violence on the unit that needs to be addressed (see Chapter 4 for additional information)
- Staff who are suffering from compassion fatigue or empathy burnout
- The absence of regular breaks and mealtimes
- Lack of support from the management team
- Staff who do not feel their input is valued or considered
- The absence of or limited teamwork
- Lack of adequate supplies, resources, and/or unhealthy work schedules

Tackling issues like these must occur first and *then* patient experience training can follow.

Because the triage nurse often sets the tone for the patient experience, special consideration should be given to the unique needs of the staff working in the triage area. The triage nurse needs to maintain positive energy while utilizing critical thinking skills; thus, rest breaks are essential. If your facility is not doing these things already, consider implementation of the following:

- A break nurse or a systematic plan to ensure the triage nurse receives regular rest, meal, and bathroom breaks
- Shorter shifts in triage (e.g., 4 or 6 hours)

Most individuals find maintaining a welcoming smile and positive attitude for an entire 12-hour triage shift to be extremely difficult; thus, shorter shifts, particularly at triage, are encouraged. *Remember: The first impression is often a lasting impression.*

Positive Staff Recognition

Programs that encourage other staff, patients, or visitors to acknowledge a person who delivers exceptional service are recommended. Recognition for a job well done praises the meaningful work, encourages a person to repeat the positive behavior, and promotes a healthier work environment. In addition, the *purpose* behind the work is celebrated. The recognition can be given to a staff member caught in the act of delivering top-notch care, having a heartfelt interaction with a patient or family member, or going above and beyond expected service. Ideas for recognizing others include:

- Use of a "hot compliments" board where others (e.g., patients, visitors, or staff) can share positive words about one staff member or the team as a whole
- "Caught ya" cards (e.g., movie tickets, coffee card, handwritten note) that are immediately given to a staff member caught in the act of providing exceptional service
- Posting positive patient satisfaction survey comments or letters from patients and family members where staff can view them
- Sending a personal, handwritten note to the home of the staff member

Honoring one staff member at a time builds team cohesiveness, supports a positive work environment, and encourages other staff to recognize the excellent work of their colleagues. In time, every team member will make the effort to acknowledge others. Only one person is needed to begin the process of creating a happier, healthier work environment. Is that staff member you?

Training for Service Excellence

During patient experience training, staff should gain a clear understanding of who their customers are. Customers in a healthcare facility extend far beyond the patient to encompass visitors, physicians, other employees, pharmaceutical representatives, and even the pizza delivery person, to name just a few. The ED is often the hospital's point-of-entry; thus, the triage team interacts with many individuals entering the facility. Patient experience training should include:

- Understanding the difference between customers and patients
- Scripting during key moments of truth (e.g., lost patient belongings or lab specimen)
- Service recovery efforts (e.g., rectifying a poor experience)

Giving staff the tools needed to deliver a positive patient experience is essential. Training can occur via the following:

- A formalized live program with lecture and discussion
- Self-paced online education
- Simulation training with case scenarios
- Observation of staff who frequently receive positive comments

Patient experience training needs to include team members throughout the continuum of care. Anyone who comes in contact with customers or patients within the facility requires training. Included in this group are:

- Direct care providers (e.g., registered nurses, licensed vocational/practical nurses, medical providers, paramedics, unlicensed personnel)
- Ancillary staff, including members from radiology, laboratory, dietary, security, and environmental services
- Administrative team members
- Volunteers

SCRIPTING

Scripting is a common catchword in healthcare today. You may be thinking, "Why scripting? Do I really need to be told what to say?" Chances are you do an excellent job in responding to questions. However, having *the right words at the most appropriate time* can make the difference in meeting patient and family needs; thus, having a few scripts available that can address certain situations is important. Scripting helps customers feel positive about the service received and has been shown to decrease the frequency with which patients leave before being seen by a medical provider. The scenarios that follow are examples of common situations that arise in the triage setting. Many other scripts can be developed that speak to the needs of common questions and concerns of your customers.

Wait Times

Scenario: An ambulatory patient who arrives at your facility encounters a WR with standing room only. As the triage nurse, you can anticipate the patient's first question.

- *The question:* How long will I have to wait?
- *What you may be thinking:* "Don't you see the 50 people sitting in the WR and lying on the floor? Didn't you hear the sirens and see the three ambulances that pulled up when you did? At the rate patients are arriving, you may wait 6, 8, or maybe even 12 hours."
- *Why you do not say what you are thinking:* Giving information about long wait times could be interpreted as coercion. Encouraging a patient to leave before receiving a medical screening exam (MSE) can lead to an Emergency Medical Treatment and Active Labor Act (EMTALA) violation, costing the facility a $50,000 fine. (See Chapter 8 for additional information.)
- *A good response:* "I wish I could give you a time, but it depends on so many factors. Patients are not seen in the order of arrival but rather based on the severity of their condition, with potentially

life-threatening conditions given the highest priority. If someone arrives in active labor nearly ready to deliver, they will be seen first." Often, lower acuity patients who believe their medical condition is a high priority understand that a woman in labor will likely be a higher treatment priority. Providing this example eliminates all lower acuity presentations (including women, men, children, and the elderly) and is rarely disputed by the waiting patient!

Directions

Scenario: A man arrives at ED triage looking for his wife, who has been transferred to the ICU.

- *The question:* How do I get to the ICU?
- *What you may be thinking:* "Does this man really think I have time to explain directions? I have ten people waiting to be triaged!"
- *Why you do not say what you are thinking:* The work you have to do is the least of this man's concerns, as his wife is critically ill.
- *A good response:* "Let me get someone to escort you so we can get you to your wife as quickly as possible." Escorting people to their destination gives a feeling of caring and compassion and lessens anxiety during times of stress.

Drinks

Scenario: A woman arrives complaining of left upper quadrant pain after a fall from a bicycle.

- *The question:* Can I have a cup of water while I wait?
- *What you may be thinking:* "Nope! Absolutely not! No way! I see a potential surgery in your future!"
- *Why you do not say what you are thinking:* Simply giving an answer of no to a patient comes off as rude, insensitive, and controlling.
- *A good response:* "I would love to get you a glass of water once we make sure your symptoms are not too serious. Your health is our top priority." Patients appreciate your concern for them, and an explanation of *why* they should not drink fluid is important.

Status Improves While Waiting

Scenario: Parents arrive with a child who has a temperature of 104°F (40°C). Acetaminophen is given at triage and the parents and child wait to be seen by a provider. While waiting, the temperature decreases to 100.1°F (38.4°C).

- *The question:* My son is feeling better so I am thinking about taking him home and seeing his pediatrician tomorrow. What do you think?

- *What you may be thinking:* "The kid looks fine, acts fine, and if he were mine, I would want to take him home too!"
- *Why you do not say what you are thinking:* You never want to downplay a patient condition. If the parents take the child home before the MSE and the child has a seizure, unidentified meningitis, or other concerning diagnosis, the child may have a poor outcome, posing a serious liability risk to both you and the facility.
- *A good response:* "I am glad he is feeling better, but I would really like to have him seen by a medical provider so we can make sure the cause of the fever is nothing of concern. I will feel better if we get him checked out and I bet you will too."

COMMUNICATION

Communication is an essential component in making customers happy. People presenting to triage are seeking *information and answers* to medical signs and symptoms. Providing information in terms that are understandable to the individual is critical. Some facilities hand out an "itinerary" upon the patient's arrival that sets the tone for the visit. The itinerary may include:

- An explanation of realistic expectations for the visit
- Rationale of why a first-come, first-served system is not utilized
- Explanations regarding wait times
- Purpose of a medical provider in triage
- When and how diagnostic testing may occur
- Why patients move between different rooms and departments
- A signature from each staff member delivering care (e.g., nurses, medical providers, and unlicensed personnel)

Consider handing out business cards to your patients or their family members. Many facilities will not supply employee business cards, but this practice is something you can do to go the extra mile. The initials after your name are often a great conversation piece with patients and visitors, especially if you hold a national certification in your area of specialty.

Fast Facts

- Be aware that simply saying the correct words means nothing if the nonverbal communication does not match the spoken words.
- Do not read from a script word for word. Rather, know the key ideas of the script and deliver the message in your own words with emotion and sincerity.
- Provide information and reassurance!

ROUNDING

Rounding in the waiting room (WR) should be a routine element of caring for patients. Depending on the facility, the role may be filled by the triage nurse, charge nurse, unlicensed personnel, or a patient advocate team member. Rounding can include:

- Checking for WR cleanliness
- Seeking answers to questions for patients and family members
- Ensuring magazines are available and the television is set to age-appropriate channels
- Increasing awareness of individuals in the WR (e.g., knowing who the patients are and who the visitors are, since you may find someone who is seeking care and never got registered or did not receive a rapid triage assessment on arrival)
- Providing a verbal update to those waiting regarding the status of the department (e.g., ED patient admissions going to the in-patient floor soon, additional staff just came on shift)

Some staff are not comfortable speaking loudly above the WR crowd. Additionally, the layout of the WR may make a one-time announcement difficult for all to hear. Regardless of the situation, communication with those waiting is imperative. Addressing multiple small groups of people can be effective as well. Many people in the WR fear the unknown. The unknown could be a diagnosis, the facility process, or the wait time. Be creative. The point is to *communicate* with those in the WR and let them know you care. However, maintaining patient privacy for specific patient-related concerns is a must.

REASSESSMENTS

Prolonged wait times can lead to changes in a patient presentation. The importance of reassessments utilizing critical thinking, guidelines (see Chapter 9), and the facility policy cannot be overstated. Reassessments may include:

- Vital signs
- Pain assessment
- Determining effectiveness of previously administered medication (e.g., fever control following acetaminophen or ibuprofen, blood glucose level after orange juice is given for hypoglycemia, pain level after an oral analgesic is administered)

Reassessment provides an additional opportunity to update patients about their status, answer questions, and give additional reassurance. Many nurses feel overwhelmed at triage and the thought of reassessing waiting patients seems impossible. However, measures to safeguard patient safety while limiting personal liability at triage are essential. Develop a facility plan to support reassessments (e.g., consider patient flow, who will reassess, and how frequently based on triage acuity level) while demonstrating concern for the patient's right to privacy.

Fast Facts

- Patients assigned a midlevel triage acuity (e.g., level 3 on a five-level scale) who wait for treatment may experience a change in medical condition. When a change in the patient's medical condition goes unnoticed, rapid deterioration may occur. Therefore, ongoing reassessment of waiting patients is critical!
- Do not let your guard down with any waiting patient!

SERVICE RECOVERY

Service recovery programs are vital when an interaction with a customer takes an undesirable turn. Staff should quickly and honestly identify the patient or visitor having a poor experience and take measures to make things better. Sometimes bringing another staff member into the situation to explain the mishap can be helpful. Owning up to an error, whether you were personally responsible for the mistake or not, can be extremely difficult to do. However, the reality is that healthcare is a service industry; thus, creating positive customer experiences is essential.

Negative Patient Experiences

Service recovery may be needed in circumstances like the following:

- The patient misunderstood the wait time frames and plan of care.
- The patient's blood tests were lost in transit to the lab.
- The required diagnostic x-ray was never ordered.
- The triage nurse stated he or she would return to the WR to escort the family member to the patient but failed to return.

Negative customer experiences should be seen as an opportunity. Steps can be taken to address the following:

- Process failures
- Communication hurdles
- Misunderstandings

Maintaining a service recovery log, and reflecting on the experiences and service recovery efforts can provide good information for future problem resolution. Does the same problem occur on the same shift routinely? Are family members always left to linger in the WR because of lack of staff who can escort them to their loved one? Efforts to identify patterns where service recovery was required should be made so the root cause can be addressed.

Resolving the Negative Experience

First and foremost, the error or negative experience should be resolved as soon as possible. In the event blood tests were lost in transit to the lab, the patient's blood specimen should be redrawn as rapidly as possible and hand delivered to the lab. After a sincere apology by the staff member for the delay, an additional service recovery effort can be initiated and may include:

- Providing a free meal in the cafeteria
- Coordinating the delivery of flowers to the patient's hospital room or home
- Giving a small gift card that can be used at the cafeteria or gift shop
- Acknowledgment from the charge nurse or management team
- Follow-up phone call the next day

EVALUATING SERVICE EXCELLENCE EFFORTS

Reflecting on patient experience practices and efforts should be ongoing in every facility. Gathering benchmark data regarding service delivery efforts before, during, and after patient experience training is important. This evaluation should occur both continually and at frequent, regular intervals. Comparing benchmark data during different time frames reveals information about attainment of preidentified metric goals and helps determine areas for improvement. Processes that enhance patient safety and patient satisfaction often improve staff satisfaction. The cycle of happier staff resulting in happier patients leads to a better environment for all.

8

Legal Concerns in Triage Nursing

Deb Jeffries

Emergency healthcare is saturated with potential legal pitfalls that are nowhere more obvious than during the ED triage process. The triage nurse must be knowledgeable about a vast array of clinical presentations, be able to think critically, and rapidly and accurately prioritize incoming patients—all while maintaining excellent customer service skills. In addition to this abbreviated list of triage nurse qualifications, the nurse must be knowledgeable about the legal expectations of ED triage. These expectations stem from governmental bodies and regulatory agencies such as the state board of nursing. The individual nurse must know what these requirements are, as defined by these entities, before a challenging situation arises.

Upon conclusion of this chapter, you will be able to:

1. State governmental and regulatory requirements affecting ED triage.
2. Identify patient's rights regarding privacy and consent.
3. Discuss high-risk legal considerations at triage.

EMERGENCY MEDICAL TREATMENT AND ACTIVE LABOR ACT

Emergency Medical Treatment and Active Labor Act (EMTALA), known as the "antidumping statute," was enacted in 1986 as part of the Consolidated Omnibus Budget Reconciliation Act of 1985 (COBRA). Often referred to as the "unfunded federal mandate,"

EMTALA responded to an ugly chapter in the history of emergency care in the United States: the "dumping" of the poor and often disenfranchised onto public hospitals. As a result of these actions by individual hospitals and staff, some patients died and poor fetal outcomes occurred as people were turned away from a handful of EDs because of their inability to pay. Out of this context, EMTALA was born. EMTALA mandates that every patient receives:

- A medical screening exam (MSE)
- Necessary stabilizing medical treatment
- An appropriate transfer to a higher level of care if necessary

Who Can Perform an MSE?

EMTALA legislation allows for a physician or a qualified medical person (QMP), identified by the facility, to perform the MSE.

Qualified Medical Person

- The hospital must formally determine who can perform the MSE.
- This must be defined in a document approved by the governing board of the hospital.
- Those designated must be identified in the hospital bylaws or in rules and regulations governing the medical staff.
- It is *not* acceptable for the medical director to make informal designations of who may perform the MSE (Centers for Medicare and Medicaid Services [CMS], 2010, 2012).

EMTALA does not specifically define (outside the conscripts just discussed) who can perform the MSE.

A hospital must formally determine who is qualified to perform the initial medical screening examinations, i.e., qualified medical person. While it is permissible for a hospital to designate a non-physician practitioner as the qualified medical person, the designated non-physician practitioner must be set forth in a document that is approved by the governing board of the hospital. (CMS, 2012, p. 5)

Fast Facts

- According to the Centers for Medicare and Medicaid Services, the MSE is anything and everything that is necessary to determine whether or not the patient has an emergency medical condition (EMC).
- An EMC is any presentation with acute symptoms of *sufficient severity* that if medical care was not provided, the patient (including those not yet born) would be at risk for serious injury or death. Symptoms of sufficient severity include *pain*.

EMTALA Pitfalls

Most ED triage nurses realize that EMTALA means that every person seeking medical care at an ED in the United States has the rights presented in this chapter. A few other stipulations include:

- Accurate documentation should be initiated for every person who presents for care, including patients who decide not to remain for treatment.
- A potential EMTALA violation exists if you *suggest* that a patient should seek care elsewhere.
- Federal law (EMTALA) supersedes state law every time.
- EMTALA applies to every hospital that has a dedicated ED and accepts Medicare funding.
- Signs must be posted informing patients of their rights.
- Signs must be provided in language(s) most common to the community seeking care.
- Hospital property includes the area within 250 yards of the building (CMS, 2010, 2012).

Fast Facts

- *Scenario:* A child is brought to the ED by a parent because of a runny nose, ear pain, and fever. The child is in no acute distress. The triage nurse tells the parent, "Your child is doing very well. To be seen quicker, there is a pediatric urgent care just across the street." Suggesting that patients seek care elsewhere is an EMTALA violation.
- The MSE or treatment *should never be delayed* to inquire about the patient's ability to pay.

CONSENT TO TREATMENT

Knowing the laws and requirements that are applicable in your facility is imperative. There are four types of consent:

- *Expressed consent:* A competent person gives consent for treatment.
- *Implied consent:* Threat to life or limb exists and the person is unable to give consent.
- *Involuntary consent:* An incompetent person refuses to consent. Competence is determined by a medical provider based on a variety of factors. Our responsibility is to thoroughly document the subjective and objective data and all interactions with the patient. *Documentation is critical!*

- *Informed consent:* Consent is given by a competent individual for a specific procedure. In some jurisdictions this consent is to be obtained by a physician.

Competent patients who are of an age and circumstance at which they can consent to treatment have the right to determine what care they will receive (Emergency Nurses Association [ENA], 2007; Hammond & Zimmermann, 2013; Howard & Steinmann, 2010).

Special Considerations Regarding Consent

Scenario: A 16-year-old girl presents to triage requesting treatment for a sexually transmitted disease but does not want her parents notified. Does she have the right to consent for her own treatment?

In most states the answer is yes. However, you must be certain of the laws regarding minors seeking care for themselves. In many states minors are allowed to seek care if it relates to pregnancy, sexually transmitted diseases, substance abuse, and methods of birth control. However, the age of consent varies from state to state and country to country. Minors who are legally emancipated may consent for their own care. Emancipation rules vary by area, so be familiar with the requirements where you practice.

Fast Facts

You are responsible for knowing the applicable laws in your state or country as well as corresponding policies at the facility in which you practice.

ACRONYMS FOR PATIENTS WHO LEAVE PRIOR TO DISCHARGE

A number of acronyms are bandied about when discussing patients who leave before they are discharged home by a provider. These terms are *not* synonymous:

- *Left without treatment (LWT):* Patients leave before or after triage.
- *Left without being seen (LWBS):* Patients leave after triage but before seeing a provider.
- *Left prior to the MSE (LPMSE):* Patients leave before or after triage but before the MSE is initiated.
- *Left before treatment complete (LBTC):* Patients leave after treatment is initiated by the provider but before formal disposition.
- *Against medical advice (AMA):* Patients leave against the advice of the provider (a subset of LBTC). By definition, this refers only to those who have been advised of the risk associated with leaving and who choose to leave regardless of those risks (Welch et al., 2011).

Although many factors influence a patient's decision to stay or leave, two of the most significant factors are the wait time and communication (or lack thereof). Almost half of those who leave would stay if comfort measures had been offered (Johnson, Myers, Wineholt, Pollack, & Kusmierz, 2009; Vierheller, 2013).

When a person leaves before the MSE is completed, an increased risk for a poor patient outcome exists. According to one study, approximately half of those who leave without being seen by a provider seek care elsewhere in the following 24 hours (Vierheller, 2013). Every effort must be made to encourage patients to stay, even when the department is at maximum capacity and the staff feel overwhelmed. When patients communicate that they want to leave, sometimes a simple inquiry as to *why* they want to leave can provide enough information to address the specific issue.

Remember you absolutely *cannot* suggest to patients that they should seek care elsewhere, and under EMTALA a log of *all* patients who present to the ED for care must be recorded regardless of whether they choose to stay. Our responsibility begins the moment that we become aware that the patient is seeking emergency care. The fact that a person has not yet received an MSE does *not* change our responsibility or the fact that the person is a patient!

HEALTH INSURANCE PORTABILITY AND ACCOUNTABILITY ACT

The Health Insurance Portability and Accountability Act of 1996 (HIPAA) is another federal mandate. So much of what we have heard since 1996 regarding HIPAA is not about the mainstay of the legislation, which was designed to combat healthcare fraud and abuse, but about the requirements to protect and ensure patient confidentiality in regard to *any individually identifiable health information*. This practice is known as *protecting personal health information (PHI)* (Hammond & Zimmermann, 2013; Howard & Steinmann, 2010). Protecting this information can be daunting during the triage process, and many ED nurses have the perception that it is not only difficult but rather impossible. This perception comes from a distorted view that confidentiality is based upon physical plant parameters when, instead, body behavior and actions of the individual obtaining the information are the driving factors.

Meeting HIPAA Privacy Requirements

We can meet HIPAA privacy requirements when interacting with patients by doing the following:

- Lowering our voice
- Moving physically closer to the patient

- When necessary, asking the patient to take a few steps away from others (including those accompanying the patient)

Although this is effective most of the time, there may be instances when we do have to inquire about the reason for the visit within the potential hearing of another. For example, as we immediately expedite the care of an individual arriving by private vehicle who is cyanotic with altered level of consciousness, another person *might* overhear an inquiry directed toward obtaining information from the patient's family. Our responsibility to patients and their families is to ensure *patient safety* through the initiation of any necessary immediate interventions. Every possible effort to maintain patient confidentiality should occur, but we cannot compromise patient safety.

Fast Facts

When in doubt about legal issues, consult with risk management.

REPORTABLE CONDITIONS AND EVENTS

Although reportable conditions and events vary from one jurisdiction to another, knowing what is reportable and what is not in your geographical area is imperative to your role as the triage nurse. Commonly reportable conditions in most states include:

- Elder abuse
- Sexual assault and rape
- Suicide
- Assault with weapons
- Stab wounds
- Injury from explosives
- Gunshot wounds
- Homicide
- Sexually transmitted infections
- Child abuse
- Certain communicable diseases (e.g., tuberculosis)
- Injury, death, or illness from a medical device

What is important to note is that privacy laws do not apply to legally defined reportable conditions or events. For example, if a patient presents to the ED with a gunshot wound and the triage nurse calls local law enforcement and provides the patient's name, address, and date of birth, the nurse has *not* committed a HIPAA violation by providing protected patient information, because this event is a reportable condition.

References

Centers for Medicare and Medicaid Services. (2010). *CMS manual system, Pub. 100-07, State operations provider certification*. Retrieved from http://www.cms.gov/Regulations-and-Guidance/Guidance/Transmittals/downloads/R60SOMA.pdf

Centers for Medicare and Medicaid Services. (2012). *State operations manual, Appendix V-Interpretive guidelines-Responsibilities of Medicare participating hospitals in emergency cases*. Retrieved from http://www.cms.gov/Regulations-and-Guidance/Guidance/Manuals/Downloads/som107ap_v_emerg.pdf

Emergency Nurses Association. (2007). *Emergency nursing core curriculum* (6th ed.). St. Louis, MO: Saunders.

Hammond, B. B., & Zimmermann, P. G. (Eds.). (2013). *Sheehy's manual of emergency care* (7th ed.). St. Louis, MO: Mosby.

Howard, P. K., & Steinmann, R. A. (Eds.). (2010). *Sheehy's emergency nursing principles and practice* (6th ed.). St. Louis, MO: Mosby.

Johnson, M., Myers, S., Wineholt, J., Pollack, M., & Kusmierz, A. L. (2009). Patients who leave the emergency department without being seen. *Journal of Emergency Nursing, 35*(2), 105–108. doi:10.1016/j.jen.2008.05.006

Vierheller, C. C. (2013). Evaluating left without being seen and against medical advice departures in a rural emergency department. *Journal of Emergency Nursing, 39*(1), 67–71. doi:10.1016/j.jen.2012.07.020

Welch, S. J., Asplin, B. R., Stone-Griffith, S., Davidson, S. J., Augustine, J., & Schuur, J. (2011). Emergency department operational metrics, measures and definitions: Results of the Second Performance Measures and Benchmarking Summit. *Annals of Emergency Medicine, 58*(1), 33–40. doi:10.1016/j.annemergmed.2010.08.040

III

Nursing Essentials for Effective Triage

9

Triage Acuity Scales

Deb Jeffries

A triage acuity level refers to the potential severity of a patient's illness or injury. Assigning a correct acuity level is one of the most important responsibilities of the triage nurse, because the prioritization of the patient determines and sets the trajectory of care for the entire patient stay. Therefore, the acuity level assigned must be an accurate reflection of the patient's condition at the time of triage. The goal of all triage acuity scales is to appropriately and accurately determine priority of care. This chapter introduces the more commonly used triage acuity scales, including the Emergency Severity Index (ESI), Canadian Triage and Acuity Scale (CTAS), Australasian Triage Scale (ATS), and Manchester Triage System (MTS).

Upon conclusion of this chapter, you will be able to:

1. Understand the significance of standardization of triage acuity scales.
2. Identify three factors that lead to mistriage.
3. List four commonly used triage acuity scales.

TRIAGE ACUITY: OVERVIEW

EDs have historically used triage scales or rating systems that were highly subjective, with little to no research as to their reliability and validity. Today, valid and reliable five-level triage scales (ESI and

Table 9.1

Comparing Triage Systems

Level	5-Level Systems	4-Level Systems	3-Level Systems	2-Level Systems
1	Resuscitation	Life-threatening		
2	Emergent	Emergent	Emergent	Emergent
3	Urgent	Urgent	Urgent	
4	Nonurgent	Nonurgent	Nonurgent	Nonemergent
5	Referred			

Source: Buettner, J. (2017). *Fast Facts for the ER Nurse* (3rd ed.). New York, NY: Springer Publishing.

CTAS) are used almost exclusively in the United States as well as elsewhere across the globe. In addition to ESI and CTAS, there are other five-level triage scales used globally, including but not limited to ATS and MTS. Each of these scales will be briefly reviewed.

Nurses have often lacked formal education related not only to the use of triage acuity scales but also to the triage process as a whole. Unfortunately, just having a nursing license and being alive continue to be the only qualifications required by some facilities for a nurse to be assigned to the triage role. This is a dangerous practice and the reader is encouraged to review the Emergency Nurses Association's Position Statement *Triage Qualifications and Competency* to gain insight into best practice regarding triage qualifications and competency. *Regardless of the specific triage acuity scale used, nurses must receive comprehensive education regarding the use of that scale.* Appropriate use of a valid and reliable five-level triage acuity scale provides discrimination between acuity levels and allows the nurse to safely determine who can and cannot wait for care (Table 9.1).

Fast Facts

- Nurses providing care at the stretcher-side can attest to the complexity of the patients seen in most EDs today. For the triage nurse, assigning the correct acuity level is first and foremost a patient safety issue.
- Assigning a correct acuity level can help staff obtain the resources needed to provide appropriate and effective patient care. However, this can only be a reality if we use a common language that communicates to strategic leaders how sick the patients really are.

MISTRIAGE

Mistriage is the assigning of a triage acuity level that is higher or lower than is warranted by the patient's presentation.

What Causes Mistriage?

A number of factors contribute to mistriage, including:

- Lack of education
- Inexperience
- Empathy burnout (Triage First Inc., 2018)

Avoiding Mistriage

Mistriage can be avoided by ensuring that:

- Nurses are educated in the triage process and the specific acuity scale being used.
- Only experienced, educated nurses are assigned to the triage role.
- Only the scale-specific criteria are used when determining acuity (Gilboy, Tanabe, Travers, & Rosenau, 2011).

Fast Facts

Although assigning either a higher or a lower acuity level than is indicated for the patient is mistriage, the chance of harming the patient by selecting the higher level is unlikely. The downfall of assigning higher levels when not indicated is using resources and occupying beds unnecessarily. However, the patient can potentially deteriorate by choosing the lower level. Triage nurses should use a valid and reliable five-level triage acuity scale and always act with the best interest of the patient in mind.

SPECIFIC TRIAGE ACUITY SCALES

The following discussion is a brief introduction to the more commonly used valid and reliable triage scales, including ESI, CTAS, ATS, and MTS. The intricate details of each triage scale cannot be covered in the limited number of pages contained in this book (and we need to be mindful of copyright issues); therefore, websites are provided to access additional information. To use these scales effectively, additional comprehensive training is required.

Emergency Severity Index

ESI is a well-researched five-level triage acuity scale with strong interrater reliability that is used extensively in the United States as well as in other countries. As it is an algorithm-driven scale, the nurse begins with every patient as a *potential* level 1 acuity and then moves down the algorithm when the patient does not meet specific criteria. For lower level acuities, ESI involves considering the number of resources (x-rays, laboratory tests, electrocardiograms, etc.) that the patient requires for the provider to make a disposition based upon what is "prudent and customary" care (Gilboy, Tanabe, Travers, & Rosenau, 2011, p. 32) as well as danger zone vital signs. ESI encompasses both adult and pediatric presentations in *The Emergency Severity Index (ESI): A Triage Tool for Emergency Department Care, Version 4. Implementation Handbook 2012 Edition*. This handbook can be obtained from the Agency for Healthcare Research and Quality by calling 1-800-358-9295 or by emailing AHRQPubs@ahrq.hhs.gov. A downloadable version of the handbook is available at www.ahrq.gov.

Canadian Triage and Acuity Scale

CTAS is also a well-researched five-level triage acuity scale used worldwide for both adult and pediatric patient populations. This scale allows for the assigning of acuity based upon the chief complaint and associated signs and symptoms along with the consideration of modifiers.

Modifiers are physiological and subjective considerations and are classified as either first order modifiers (e.g., vital signs, pain severity, mechanism of injury), which apply to many complaints, or second order modifiers (e.g., hypoglycemia), which are more specifically related to fewer complaints. This acuity scale provides reassessment time frame guidelines. CTAS implementation guidelines and subsequent revisions can be obtained at www.caep.ca/resources/ctas#support.

Australasian Triage Scale

The ATS is a valid and reliable five-category scale that is used in New Zealand and Australia. This scale was developed with the goal of matching the patient's clinical urgency with timelines of care by considering how long a patient should wait for assessment and treatment from the time of his or her arrival. The ATS uses a conceptual question to drive the acuity designation by asking, "This patient should wait for medical assessment and treatment no longer than ..." (Australasian College for Emergency Medicine, 2013a, p. 1). Clinical descriptors assist the nurse in determining the acuity level. For example, some category 1 clinical descriptors include the following (Australasian College for Emergency Medicine, 2013b):

- Cardiac or respiratory arrest or both
- Imminent risk to airway
- Extreme respiratory distress
- Unresponsive or responds to pain only
- Blood pressure less than 80 mmHg in adults
- Child or infant in severe shock

Additional information and guidelines regarding the use of the ATS can be accessed at https://acem.org.au/getmedia/484b39f1-7c99-427b-b46e-005b0cd6ac64/P06-Policy-on-the-ATS-Jul-13-v04.aspx and https://www.cena.org.au.

Manchester Triage System

The MTS is a valid and reliable five-level triage acuity scale developed in the United Kingdom and widely used all over Europe. This acuity system uses an algorithm approach with over 50 detailed flowcharts. An example of a flowchart can be viewed at tinyurl.com/mw4qhqr. The triage nurse chooses a flowchart based upon the patient's presenting complaint. The nurse then makes the acuity decision based upon signs and symptoms, also known as discriminators, as they relate to the flowchart chosen. General discriminators can be viewed at tinyurl.com/pvvnn6f. The MTS core text by the Manchester Triage Group (Mackway-Jones, Marsden, & Windle, 2014) provides additional information about this acuity scale.

Fast Facts

Not all patients fit into our nice, neat acuity categories. However, when the acuity scale criteria are used, most of the time you will be able to determine the appropriate acuity level.

A Few Final Thoughts

As noted earlier, this survey of the five-level triage acuity scale is merely a brief introduction. *Any* emergency nurse with the responsibility of assigning an acuity designation must be thoroughly familiar with the specific criteria of the scale being used. To accomplish this, *education is a must.*

Another often-debated issue surrounding triage acuity designations is whether, once assigned, the triage acuity should be changed based upon a change in patient status or because a colleague disagrees with the original acuity assigned. The answer to this question is a resounding "No!" Once assigned, the original triage acuity *does not change*. (Hint: The key word is *triage acuity*; it is not a treatment area acuity.) The debate relating to this issue often surrounds established facility-specific policies for reassessment based upon the triage acuity.

Fast Facts

A patient "acuity level" is rarely static. Patients can improve or deteriorate, and therefore an acuity level may be *updated* based upon the patient's current status. However, the acuity level assigned to the patient at the time of the triage assessment *does not change*.

References

Australasian College for Emergency Medicine. (2013a). *Guidelines on the implementation of the Australasian triage scale in emergency department (version 3)*. Retrieved from https://acem.org.au/getmedia/51dc74f7-9ff0-42ce-872a-0437f3db640a/G24_04_Guidelines_on_Implementation_of_ATS_Jul-16.aspx

Australasian College for Emergency Medicine. (2013b). *Policy on the Australasian triage scale (version 4)*. Retrieved from https://acem.org.au/getmedia/484b39f1-7c99-427b-b46e-005b0cd6ac64/P06-Policy-on-the-ATS-Jul-13-v04.aspx

Gilboy, N., Tanabe, T., Travers, D., & Rosenau, A. M. (2011). *Emergency severity index (ESI): A triage tool for emergency department care, version 4. Implementation handbook 2012 edition* (AHRQ Publication No. 12-0014). Rockville, MD: Agency for Healthcare Research and Quality. Retrieved from http://www.ahrq.gov/sites/default/files/wysiwyg/professionals/systems/hospital/esi/esihandbk.pdf

Mackway-Jones, K., Marsden, J., & Windle, J. (Eds.). (2014). *Emergency triage: Manchester triage group* (3rd ed.). Chichester: John Wiley.

Triage First, Inc. (2018). ED Triage: Comprehensive Course. Asheville, NC: Author.

10

Triage Documentation

Rebecca S. McNair

Triage is a process, not a place. Therefore, triage entails the process of patient throughput from the point of entry to patient disposition and transfer of care to the next provider in the emergency treatment area. Documentation of this process is mandatory and serves multiple purposes. These purposes include creating an archive of the patient with the goal of ensuring quality patient care, proving adherence to professional standards of care and organizational policies and procedures, and advocating for the patient through clear communication between care providers. Many documentation components are necessary for a comprehensive triage assessment, although some of this documentation may occur at the bedside if immediate bedding is implemented following the rapid triage assessment (See Chapter 6 for additional information on this topic.) This chapter focuses on the essentials of good triage documentation.

Upon conclusion of this chapter, you will be able to:

1. Recognize a systematic approach for the collection and recording of necessary triage data in the patient medical record.
2. State one mnemonic to guide the subjective component of a triage assessment.
3. State all elements of the objective component of a triage assessment.
4. Identify key elements required for meeting best practice in triage documentation.

ESSENTIAL COMPONENTS OF GOOD DOCUMENTATION

The hallmarks of good documentation include *brevity* and *clarity*. To be both brief and clear, one must use a *systematic approach*, which involves performing the assessment and concordant documentation in essentially the same manner every time, using a SOAP (*Subjective, Objective, Assessment, Plan*) format. The essential components of good documentation for a comprehensive (2–5 minutes) triage assessment include the following.

Arrival Time

- Actual time of initial patient arrival to the facility

Time Seen by the Triage Nurse

- Actual time at which rapid and comprehensive triage assessments begin (see Chapter 6 for additional information)

Documentation of Subjective Triage Assessment

- *Symptom-driven chief complaint:* This is the *reason for the patient's visit.*
- *Subjective line of questioning (LOQ)*
- *Medications, allergies* (agent *and* specific adverse reactions)
- *Pertinent mandatory screenings:* Mandatory screenings at triage vary according to organizations (e.g., fall risk, intimate partner violence, nutritional screen, etc.); thus, follow your facility protocol.
- *Pain assessment:* This parameter of the patient's subjective experience *must* be noted in every visit and includes physical, psychological, and social distress.

Fast Facts

- Patients may misinterpret their symptoms. If a patient presents with a complaint of migraine headache, the triage nurse is responsible to *ask* the patient what symptoms he or she is having and then *document* the chief complaint in symptom form, such as *headache, photophobia, and nausea*. When using electronic medical records with prepopulated chief complaint fields, consider the option to provide a free text note of the chief complaint if the system does not support a symptom-driven chief complaint. *Remember that it is not a nursing function to document diagnostically.*
- Never document a chief complaint by referring to an organ or structure that you cannot see (e.g., kidney pain, stomach pain, rib pain). Always ask the patient to point to the area of complaint and then document the anatomical location (e.g., RUQ [*right upper quadrant*] abdominal pain).

Documentation of Objective Triage Assessment

- General observations of body systems, including:
  - *Mode of arrival:* An ambulatory patient, mobile with use of an assistive device (e.g., cane, walker, or wheelchair) or an uneven gait (e.g., staggering, limping)
  - *Abnormal observations:* Hygiene, clothing, odor resembling alcohol on breath
  - *Respiratory status:* Respiratory rate, rhythm, effort (e.g., labored or unlabored)
  - *Neurological status:* Alert and oriented to person, time, place, and event
  - *Integumentary status:* Skin color, temperature, moisture
- Pertinent vital signs
- Pain assessment (objective observations)
- Focused physical assessment pertinent to chief complaint

Fast Facts

- The necessity of obtaining an accurate weight in *kilograms* for patients seeking medical care is well documented as many medications require weight-based dosing.
- When errors occur during the process of obtaining, documenting, and communicating a patient's weight, the dose of a medication can be dangerously incorrect. (Bailey, Gaunt, Grissinger, & Pennsylvania Patient Safety Authority, 2016)

Assessment Statement

- Acuity category or severity index rating based on a statistically valid and reliable triage acuity scale or severity index

Plan

- Any diagnostic tests and care ordered
- Disposition (initial disposition if the patient is assigned to wait, as well as treatment area disposition)

Interventions

- Diagnostics and care rendered (x-ray, ice, medications, etc.)

Evaluation

- Effectiveness of triage interventions initiated

Reassessments

- Should be recorded at appropriate intervals as dictated by the triage acuity scale, facility, or organizational guidelines, and should reflect the standard of care for each acuity category
- Should occur if a change is noted by the patient, spouse, nursing or ancillary staff

Fast Facts

- Patients interpret the word *pain* as having a very specific meaning. Try rephrasing your questions as follows: "Are you having *any discomfort* at all? Are you experiencing any unusual feelings? Can you describe those feelings?" Use the mnemonic PQRST to obtain additional information. PQRST is discussed further in the pages that follow.
- Documentation of pain must include both subjective *and* objective elements. If the patient reports a high level of pain and the nurse assigns a low triage acuity category, then supportive data must be documented to validate that lower acuity level. For example:
  - Subjective: Patient states he is "in severe pain and cannot even work"; rates pain 8 on a 0 to 10 scale
  - Objective: Patient observed laughing and walking around waiting area, talking on mobile phone

DOCUMENTATION OF AGAINST MEDICAL ADVICE, LEFT PRIOR TO TREATMENT, LEFT WITHOUT BEING SEEN, LEFT WITHOUT TREATMENT, LEFT PRIOR TO MEDICAL SCREENING EXAM

See Chapter 8 for information regarding patients' leaving before completion of care.

MNEMONICS TO GUIDE DOCUMENTATION

Mnemonics can help the triage nurse drive the line of questioning, which facilitates documentation. See Chapter 30 for more information regarding mnemonics that assist in pediatric documentation.

Mnemonic: OLD CART

Onset of symptoms (or injury—how and when did it happen)
Location of symptoms (or injury)
Duration of symptoms
Characteristics of symptoms described by patient

Aggravating factors
Relieving factors
Treatment administered before arrival and outcome

Mnemonic for Pain Assessment: PQRST

Provokes and **P**alliates
- What makes it worse? What makes it better?

Quality
- What does the pain feel like (aching, sharp, dull, pressing, stabbing, etc.)?

Region and **R**adiation
- Where is the pain located? Does it radiate to any other part of the body? (Ask the patient to point to where it hurts.)

Severity and associated **S**ymptoms
- Use of a 0 to 10 visual analog scale: 0 = none and 10 = worst pain imaginable (not the worst pain you have ever had, as some individuals have never experienced a 10 out of 10 pain)
- Mild–moderate–severe (severe pain significantly interferes with activities of daily living)
- Other pain rating scales
- Pediatric pain assessment scales

Timing and **T**emporal relations
- Onset and duration?
- Constant or intermittent pain?

KEY LINE OF QUESTIONING FOR MOTOR VEHICLE CRASH

- You were involved in a motor vehicle crash, when?
- Were you the driver or passenger?
- (If passenger) Where were you sitting in the car?
- Were you wearing a seat belt?
- Airbag? (If yes) Deployed?
- How did the crash occur?
- How fast were the vehicles traveling, approximately?
- How much damage to the vehicle(s) involved?
- Was anyone else hurt in the crash?
- How did you get out of the car?
- Where do you hurt?
- Is anything else bothering you?

Fast Facts

- Sometimes words are documented inappropriately, most likely due to confusion regarding their meaning. Knowing

(continued)

(*continued*)

> the definition behind the words you use in documentation is important. Examples of words commonly confused are *lethargic*, *drowsy*, *irritable*, and *fussy*.
> - *Lethargic* versus *drowsy: Lethargy* can be defined as unusual sleepiness, denotes a significant neurological sequela, and is evidenced by a child who cannot be easily aroused. *Drowsiness* would be used for the most common symptom after crying, or from a lack of sleep, and the child can be easily aroused.
> - *Irritable* versus *fussy: Irritability* may indicate a serious neurological event. Children who are truly irritable are unable to be consoled (by a caregiver, bottle, pacifier, or other comfort measures). Such inconsolable crying is often seen in the child who presents with meningitis. Fussy infants and children have many reasons for crying or being fussy, including discomfort, fever, anxiety, hunger, or exhaustion. (Triage First, 2018)

Websites for additional information on pain assessments include:

- The American Society for Pain Management Nursing at www.aspmn.org/Pages/default.aspx
- American Pain Society at www.americanpainsociety.org

References

Bailey, B. R., Gaunt, M. J., Grissinger, M., & Pennsylvania Patient Safety Authority. (2016). Update on medication errors associated with incorrect patient weights. *Pennsylvania Patient Safety Advisory, 13*(2), 50–57. Retrieved from http://patientsafety.pa.gov/ADVISORIES/documents/201606_50.pdf

Triage First, Inc. (2018). ED Triage Comprehensive Course. Asheville, North Carolina: Author.

11

Time-Sensitive Medical Conditions

Lynn Sayre Visser

Core measures are national initiatives used to drive quality patient care, grounded by evidence-based research, with the goal of achieving best patient outcomes. Approximately 10 core measures exist with several specifically influencing ED care. Prehospital personnel, hospital-based employees, telephone triage nurses, and urgent care staff should be aware of these measures so actions can be taken to ensure the patient receives appropriate care. Acute myocardial infarction (AMI), pneumonia, and stroke are the most common core measure presentations seen in the ED, with sepsis being a likely up-and-coming core measure.

Upon conclusion of this chapter, you will be able to:

1. Identify screening and assessment questions for core measure initiatives in the ED.
2. Describe three core measure treatment goals.
3. List key core measure nursing actions.

CORE MEASURES

Triage nurses play an important role with time-sensitive conditions often referred to as core measures. Meeting core measure timelines requires the triage nurse to be familiar with the associated criteria. Asking the right questions at the right time is essential. Consistently applying screening measures aids in appropriately identifying patients who are at risk for time-sensitive diagnoses. Early recognition leads to initiation of treatment that can greatly decrease mortality risk and enhance patient outcomes. For the purposes of this book, a basic understanding of signs and symptoms of many conditions is assumed.

ACUTE MYOCARDIAL INFARCTION

AMI can be symptomatic or asymptomatic. Early recognition is critical because mortality and morbidity rates are increased in the face of an AMI. *Remember: Time is muscle!*

Screening Questions/Assessment

Questions you will want to ask to determine the level of concern for an AMI center on the presence of the following symptoms:

- Chest pain? If the patient responds yes to an inquiry about the presence of chest pain, ask the PQRST (provokes and palliates; quality; region and radiation; severity and associated symptoms; timing and temporal relations) questions, including whether the pain radiates to the back, shoulder, arms, jaw, or neck.
- Associated shortness of breath or dyspnea?
- Epigastric pain, nausea, vomiting, or associated diaphoresis?
- Dizziness, syncopal episode(s), or chest pain unrelieved with rest?

Risk Factors for AMI

- *Modifiable risk factors:* Obesity, tobacco use, substance abuse, high cholesterol, elevated serum lipids, diabetes, hypertension, decreased physical activity, and psychosocial issues
- *Nonmodifiable risk factors:* Ethnicity, increasing age, gender (men generally more at risk than women), genetic predisposition, and family history of heart disease

Treatment Goals

Upon suspicion of an AMI, treatment should be initiated with careful consideration to mandated time frames indicated in Table 11.1.

Utilizing a core measure order set can assist staff with meeting treatment guidelines. Most likely the triage nurse will not be the one to ensure follow-through on all elements of the guidelines, but this nurse holds the key to identifying individuals who need the core measure treatment initiated. In some facilities, the triage nurse indicates the initiation of the core measure order set in the computer system or places a copy of the order set on the paper chart. This practice raises awareness to the care team.

Table 11.1

AMI Treatment Goals

Time Frame	Treatment
Within 10 minutes of arrival	ECG
Upon arrival	Aspirin
Before giving a thrombolytic	CXR
Within <30 minutes of arrival	Thrombolytic or cardiac catheterization lab
Within <90 minutes of arrival	Percutaneous coronary intervention (door to needle timeline)

AMI, acute myocardial infarction; CXR, chest x-ray.

You may be thinking, "There is no possible way I can get an ECG within the first 10 minutes at *my facility*!" Obtaining the ECG at triage can be difficult because of space constraints, but the necessity of obtaining the ECG cannot be overemphasized. The ECG can occur on a gurney, in a reclining chair, or upright if there are no other options. Some locations and physical positions may be less than optimal for both the patient and staff but flexibility (literally!) may be required to initiate the preliminary ECG.

Key Nursing Actions at Triage

- Document arrival time and use this time as "time zero" for implementing care.
- Initiate basic life support measures for airway, breathing, and circulation management.
- Obtain the ECG within the first 10 minutes of patient arrival; refer to your facility protocol.
- Initiate an ST-segment elevation myocardial infarction (STEMI) alert per protocol if applicable; a predesignated team of people come together rapidly to provide the standard of care (e.g., rapid response team, nurses, physicians, radiology, lab, pharmacy staff, critical care transport).
- Transport the patient from triage to the treatment area/team immediately by wheelchair or gurney.
- Anticipate the need for oxygen, venous access, chest x-ray (CXR), medications, and laboratory testing.
- Notify the provider of the high-acuity patient presentation.
- Flag the medical record as a time-sensitive situation to increase staff awareness.

Although you may not personally perform each intervention at triage, know your policies and advocate appropriately so the patient obtains timely care. Current guidelines for cardiac care are available from the American College of Cardiology/American Heart Association and may be retrieved from www.acc.org/guidelines.

Fast Facts

- The triage nurse plays a pivotal role in identifying individuals who potentially meet core measure criteria and ensuring that specific core measure treatment is initiated.
- Meeting the timelines with 100% efficiency not only provides quality evidence-based care and patient safety but demonstrates the ability of the hospital to follow requirements developed by the Joint Commission and the Centers for Medicare and Medicaid Services.

STROKE

A stroke, or cerebrovascular accident, is the interruption of cerebral blood flow. The onset of neurological symptoms within the past 48 hours is representative of an acute stroke. As in an AMI, recognition of a stroke is essential for reducing patient morbidity and mortality. Patients with evolving ischemic strokes lose 1.9 million neurons and 14 billion synapses per minute, aging the human brain by 3.6 years per hour (Saver, 2006). This translates to the destruction of 7.5 mi (12 km) of myelinated fibers (Saver, 2006). Every 40 seconds an American has a stroke and every 4 minutes an American dies of a stroke (Centers for Disease Control and Prevention, 2018). These alarming statistics validate the need for rapid initiation of treatment. *Remember: Time is brain tissue!*

Screening Questions/Assessment

To determine the level of concern for a possible stroke, consider whether there was sudden onset of any of the following signs and symptoms (National Stroke Association, n.d.):

- Presence of confusion, difficulty understanding others, or slurred speech?
- Visual disturbances in one or both eyes?
- Presence of one-sided arm, leg, or face weakness or numbness?
- Severe headache without known cause?
- Dizziness or difficulty walking or maintaining balance?
- Impaired physical coordination?

Finally, inquire when the patient was *last seen normal* (at his or her baseline) or "last known well" as this information is critical and will influence the treatment plan.

Risk Factors for Stroke

- *Modifiable risk factors:* High blood pressure, diabetes, atherosclerosis, high cholesterol, atrial fibrillation, circulation problems, obesity, alcohol use, tobacco use (e.g., smoking or chewing), and physical inactivity
- *Nonmodifiable risk factors:* Age, gender, race, family history, previous stroke or transient ischemic attack (TIA), and patent foramen ovale (National Stroke Association, 2014)

Treatment Goals

A patient who exhibits signs and symptoms of a stroke will need a rapid evaluation and CT scan of the head to determine the type of stroke (e.g., hemorrhagic or ischemic) and candidacy for thrombolytic therapy or other interventional treatment. The actions of the triage nurse should be the same regardless of the diagnostic outcome. Guidelines for stroke care are available from the American Heart Association/American Stroke Association in the 2018 Guidelines for the Early Management of Patients with Acute Ischemic Stroke located at stroke.ahajournals.org/content/49/3/e46.long. Table 11.2 outlines the care guidelines.

Identification of stroke patients focuses on the time the patient was *last seen normal*. Patients receive the most substantial benefit from the initiation of intravenous thrombolytic therapy when given

Table 11.2

Stroke Care Treatment Goals

Time Frame	Treatment
Within 10 minutes of arrival	Perform a triage assessment Neurological screening ED medical provider evaluation
Within 15 minutes of arrival	Activate stroke team
Within 25 minutes of arrival	Obtain CT scan of head
Within 45 minutes of arrival	Head CT interpretation
Within 60 minutes of arrival	Determine candidacy for fibrinolytics Door-to-drug time
Within 3 hours of symptom onset	Begin postfibrinolytic pathway

within the first hour of *symptom onset*, although thrombolytic therapy given up to 4.5 hours after the beginning of symptoms has significant benefits. The Cincinnati Prehospital Stroke Scale or the Los Angeles Prehospital Stroke Screen are tools that can be used at triage to rapidly assess a patient for stroke symptoms. Many facilities utilize the National Institutes of Health Stroke Scale (NIHSS), a valid and reliable clinical stroke assessment tool that determines the severity of the condition of the stroke patient and helps guide treatment. Use of this tool should *not delay* movement of the patient from triage to the treatment team. *Time is of the essence*; thus, quick identification of a potential stroke candidate and critical thinking skills at triage can significantly impact the patient outcome and possibly prevent a catastrophic permanent disability.

New research is showing incredible benefits from thrombectomy even when a patient was last seen normal up to 24 hours prior. These patients require rapid cerebral CT angiography (CTA)/CT perfusion (CTP), and MRI scans so they can receive the intervention as soon as possible. The DAWN and DEFUSE (Nogueira et al., 2018; Albers et al., 2018) trials will make these patients important to identify rapidly in the triage setting so they can be treated appropriately.

Key Nursing Actions at Triage

- Document arrival time and use this time as "time zero" for implementing care (refers to the time frames indicated in Table 11.2).
- Initiate basic life support measures for airway, breathing, and circulation management.
- Begin rapid identification of stroke signs and symptoms.
- Determine the time when the patient was last seen normal.
- Initiate a stroke alert/stroke team activation per facility protocol.
- Notify the medical provider of the high-acuity patient presentation.
- Flag the medical record as a time-sensitive situation to increase staff awareness.

PNEUMONIA

A patient who arrives with symptoms that raise suspicion of pneumonia needs a quick screening to determine if criteria exist that require expedited treatment to meet core measure timelines. Processes should be in place to capture the right candidates. Overcrowding can lead to increased wait times, and if devised systems are not adhered to, delays in treatment may occur. Timely antibiotic administration is the essential component of this core measure. *Remember: Time is multiplying organisms and increasing infection!*

Screening Questions/Assessment

When evaluating a patient for a suspicion of pneumonia, consider whether any of the following signs and symptoms are present:

- Fever, fatigue, weakness, or malaise?
- Shortness of breath, cough, or chest discomfort?
- Adventitious lung sounds?
- Vital sign abnormality, including respiratory rate greater than 20 breaths per minute, heart rate greater than 100 beats per minute (bpm), pulse oximetry less than 95% on room air, or temperature greater than 100.4°F (38°C)?

Risk Factors for Pneumonia

- Cancer, chemotherapy, or other cancer treatments; recent organ transplant; HIV; heart disease; chronic bronchitis or emphysema; nausea, vomiting, poor gag reflex, or difficulty swallowing; recent viral infection, cold symptoms, or upper respiratory tract infection; elderly, recent hospital stay, or living in a long-term-care facility; recent chest injury or surgery; prolonged bed rest

Treatment Goals

- The goal for door-to-antibiotic time is less than 6 hours (time begins to run upon patient arrival).
- Prior to antibiotics being administered, two sets of blood cultures should be obtained.
- Obtain a CXR as soon as possible after patient arrival.

Key Nursing Actions at Triage

- Document arrival time and use this time as "time zero" for implementing care.
- Initiate basic life support measures for airway, breathing, and circulation management.
- Begin rapid identification of pneumonia signs and symptoms.
- Initiate advanced triage protocols per facility policy or advocate for orders.
- Notify the provider of the time-sensitive patient presentation.
- Flag the medical record as a time-sensitive situation to increase staff awareness.

Fast Facts

Knowing core measure treatment goal timelines is an essential first step in meeting the goals! Referencing core measure order sets helps staff focus on the specific criteria and prevents missing key components.

OTHER MEASURES AND POTENTIAL UP-AND-COMING CORE MEASURES

Additional core measures, including pediatric asthma and congestive heart failure, exist. However, they do not have the same level of time sensitivity as the conditions discussed in this chapter. Please refer to www.jointcommission.org or www.qualitymeasures.ahrq.gov for additional information.

SEPSIS, SEVERE SEPSIS, AND SEPTIC SHOCK

Sepsis, severe sepsis, and septic shock are serious health concerns requiring timely, appropriate intervention. To date sepsis is not a core measure, but patient outcomes rely on time-driven care. Thus, understanding the guidelines for caring for septic patients is imperative. Additional information on this topic is available at www.survivingsepsis.org. *Remember: Time is multiplying organisms, systemic involvement, organ dysfunction, and hypoperfusion!*

Screening Questions/Assessment

Two important screening questions for sepsis exist and are listed below in Part I. Each patient presenting to your facility should be screened using the three-part process below.

Part I: Infection

Is there presence or suspicion of an infection? Is the patient taking antibiotics? If yes to either question, continue to Part II.

Part II: Systemic Inflammatory Response Syndrome (SIRS) Criteria

Determine whether the patient meets at least *two* of the criteria listed below:

- Altered mental status from the patient's baseline
- Temperature greater than 101.0°F (38.3°C) or less than 96.8°F (36°C)
- Heart rate greater than 90 bpm
- Respiratory rate greater than 20 breaths per minute
- White blood cell (WBC) count greater than 12,000/µL or WBC count less than 4,000/µL
- Hyperglycemia greater than 140 mg/dL? (Society for Critical Care Medicine, n.d.)

If criteria in both Part I and Part II are met, proceed to Part III.

Part III: Acute Organ Failure

Screening for the presence of organ dysfunction criteria at triage should also occur and includes the following (Society for Critical Care Medicine, n.d.):

- Systolic blood pressure (SBP) less than 90 mmHg or mean arterial pressure (MAP) less than 65 mmHg
- SBP decrease greater than 40 mmHg from baseline
- Lactate greater than 2 mmol/L (18.0 mg/dL)
- Platelet count less than 100,000/μL
- International normalized ratio (INR) greater than 1.5 or partial thromboplastin time (PTT) greater than 60 seconds
- Creatinine greater than 2.0 mg/dL
- Urine output less than 0.5 mL/kg/hr for 2 hours
- Increased oxygen need to maintain oxygen saturation greater than 90%

This information is important for the triage nurse, as many facilities initiate nursing protocols at triage while the patient waits for a treatment bed. Early initiation of nursing protocols may uncover the most common signs of acute organ failure. Severe sepsis is met if *both* a suspicion of infection and the presence of organ dysfunction exist.

Risk Factors for Sepsis

- Presence of a bacterial infection anywhere in the body, including the bloodstream, bones, skin, or organs; surgical wounds, burns, or decubitus ulcers; invasive lines (e.g., central lines), surgical drains, or breathing tubes
- Immunocompromised status

Treatment Goals

To be completed within 3 hours of presentation of severe sepsis, the patient should receive:

- Initial lactate level measurement
- Broad-spectrum or other antibiotic(s) administered
- Blood cultures drawn prior to antibiotics

Key Nursing Actions at Triage

- Document arrival time and use this time as "time zero" for implementing care.
- Initiate basic life support measures for airway, breathing, and circulation management.
- Recognize the potential patient in severe sepsis or septic shock.

- Use a severe sepsis screening tool to identify patients who meet criteria; the Surviving Sepsis Campaign offers a screening tool at www.survivingsepsis.org/SiteCollectionDocuments/ScreeningTool.pdf.
- Initiate a sepsis alert per facility protocol.
- Raise awareness of the patient arrival to the treatment team.
- Start advanced triage protocols per policy or advocate for medical provider treatment orders.

Fast Facts

- Be familiar with the screening criteria for a patient with a possible AMI, stroke, pneumonia, or sepsis.
- Time is heart muscle! Time is brain! Time is multiplying organisms and increasing infection! As the triage nurse, you hold the key that can be the difference between life and death. Time is of the essence!

References

Albers, G. W., Marks, M. P., Kemp, S., Christensen, S., Tsai, J. P., Ortega-Gutierrez, S., . . . Lansberg, M. G. (2018). Thrombectomy for stroke at 6 to 16 hours with selection by perfusion imaging. *New England Journal of Medicine, 378*, 708–718. doi:10.1056/NEJMoa1713973

Centers for Disease Control and Prevention. (2018). Shingles (herpes zoster). Retrieved from https://www.cdc.gov/shingles/index.html

National Stroke Association. (n.d.). Stroke resources. Retrieved from http://www.stroke.org/stroke-resources?gclid=EAIaIQobChMIuPSrpYnX2wI

National Stroke Association. (2014). *Am I at risk for a stroke?* Retrieved from http://www.stroke.org

Nogueira, R. G., Jadhav, A. P., Haussen, D. C., Bonafe, A., Budzik, R. F., Bhuva, P., . . . Jovin, T. G. (2018). Thrombectomy 6 to 24 hours after stroke with a mismatch between deficit and infarct. *New England Journal of Medicine, 378*, 11–21. doi:10.1056/NEJMoa1706442

Saver, J. (2006). Time is brain-quantified. *Journal of the American Heart Association, 37*, 263–266. doi:10.1161/01.STR.0000196957.55928.ab

Society for Critical Care Medicine. (n.d.). Evaluation for severe sepsis screening. Retrieved September 29, 2018 from http://www.survivingsepsis.org/Resources/Pages/Protocols-and-Checklists.aspx

IV

Current Trends Impacting Triage Nursing

12

Urgent Care Triage

Valerie Aarne Grossman

The purpose of urgent care centers (UCCs) is to serve the urgent medical needs of patients in a cost-effective, high-quality manner outside the more expensive hospital ED. The urgent care arena is not intended to care for emergent or high-acuity medical needs of patients. These are different settings, managed by different groups, aimed at different populations, but all with the same end goal: to provide a healthcare service to those in need in an appropriate manner. This chapter begins the discussion of the growing use of UCCs, which operate under a variety of names yet all with a similar purpose.

Upon the conclusion of this chapter, you will be able to:

1. State three benefits that UCCs offer to those seeking care.
2. Discuss the role of triage in a UCC.
3. Understand the necessity of UCCs.

BACKGROUND

UCCs began in the 1980s as a solution to the limitation of the private physician's office and the rapidly growing census of the already crowded EDs. Over the past 30 years, these centers have continued to grow in number, improve access to care, lower episodic healthcare costs (especially after-hours), and provide a wider variety of services than were initially available. Depending on the center, they may offer:

- Laboratory services
- Medication administration (e.g., influenza vaccines)
- Radiology services
- Care to patients across the age spectrum
- Drug testing
- Application of splints and casts (simple bone fractures)
- Simple laceration repair
- Administration of intravenous hydration
- Occupational health services
- School and employment physical exams

Many centers target their hours of operation to overlap peak hours of the local EDs or provide coverage when private physician offices are typically closed (e.g., weekday evenings, weekends, and holidays). Over the past decades, as many hospitals (and their EDs) have closed their doors, the number of displaced patients seeking care for their urgent health needs has increased.

STAFFING

The skill level and number of personnel working at a UCC will depend on the size and scope (facility specific), and governing agency regulations, and is tailored to the exact services offered. Staffing could include:

- Physicians
- Physician assistants
- Nurse practitioners
- Registered nurses
- Registration clerks
- Licensed practical/vocational nurses
- Patient care technicians (unlicensed)
- Radiologic or laboratory technologists or both

REGULATIONS

Regulations that a UCC may need to follow greatly vary. Each professional working in the center will have his or her own licensing guidelines to follow, and the center itself will need to comply with the governing rules under which it is credentialed. For example, if the UCC is part of a hospital setting, the center will need to comply with the Emergency Medical Treatment and Active Labor Act (EMTALA).

> **Fast Facts**
>
> The regulations under which a center will operate usually depend on the "owner" of the clinic (physician owned, hospital owned, corporation owned, etc.).

SERVICE AND SCOPE

Retail medical clinics (RMCs) are being built in national pharmacy and grocery chains. In 2012, there were over 1,000 such clinics. It is estimated that more than $4 billion annually can be saved when patients utilize the services of UCCs or RMCs instead of hospital EDs (Mann, 2014). The services delivered by each UCC or RMC may vary to meet the needs of the community, the practice vision of the owner, or the licensure of those it employs. No intention of an ongoing provider–patient relationship exists, as care is delivered on an episodic basis only.

TRIAGE

The typical UCC operates on a first-come, first-served basis, although when an acute or emergent patient walks in the door, he or she should be seen ahead of all waiting. In larger centers, a system of triage may be employed similar to the five-tier triage system used in an ED. There is no master list of appropriate patient complaints that would be cared for at a UCC, as any complaint may have a more critical underlying component. However, typical minor complaints that could be cared for at a UCC may include:

- Dental complaints
- Dysuria
- Ear pain
- Fever
- Foreign body removal
- Headache
- Medication refill
- Minor eye complaints
- Minor laceration
- Minor skin infection
- Minor trauma
- Muscle aches and pain
- Nausea, vomiting, diarrhea
- Nosebleed
- Rash
- Sexual transmitted disease

- Sore throat
- Sprains and strains
- Sunburn
- Suture removal
- Upper respiratory illness

For specific triage applications, please refer to the "red flag" patient presentation chapters in Part V of this book.

Fast Facts

Any minor complaint can easily have a complicated, hidden origin. Quickly rule out serious conditions for simple complaints or triage to a higher level of care delivery.

UCCs and RMCs play an important role in the overall delivery of healthcare in the United States. They fill the gap between scheduled appointments in a physician's practice and the overcrowded EDs, which are utilized for any health need by a large and varied population. These alternatives offer a wide range of healthcare services, at a more cost-effective rate than a hospital ED, and are often open at convenient hours and locations for those seeking care.

Reference

Mann, C. (2014). *CMCS informational bulletin: Reducing nonurgent use of emergency departments and improving appropriate care in appropriate settings*. Retrieved from http://www.medicaid.gov/Federal-Policy-Guidance/Downloads/CIB-01-16-14.pdf

13

Electronic Medical Record Considerations

Dawn Friedly Gray

Electronic medical records (EMRs) are being introduced everywhere as a result of government regulations requiring facilities to follow meaningful use guidelines and improve patient care through increased access to electronic documentation. Documentation should accurately reflect decision-making processes and support care delivery. Avoiding charting pitfalls can improve the delivery of care. Fast and accurate documentation enhances communication, improves throughput times, and leads to better patient outcomes and higher-quality care. This chapter reviews key concepts to remember regarding triage EMR documentation.

Upon conclusion of this chapter, you will be able to:

1. List three concepts you need to know about the EMR and effective triage practices.
2. State how utilizing an EMR in triage can improve patient outcomes.
3. Identify three common pitfalls of the EMR in the triage setting.

BENEFITS OF THE EMR

Triage is a process occurring at many different times and places. It is important to use your assessment skills to elicit information when determining the priority needs of the patient and avoid distraction by the structure and functionality of the EMR. Documentation should be simple and reflect the care delivered by the triage nurse.

Proper identification is essential when opening a patient's EMR. Be sure to use two patient identifiers and compare the name bracelet to the name on the EMR while asking patients who they are. You will also need to identify if the patient has special needs, cultural sensitivities, privacy concerns, religious observances, translator needs, or transgender sensitivities. Be sure to document in the chart what you learn about the special care some patients may need or require. Whether it is a sign language interpreter or the preferred gender identification, this key information is part of the foundation of patient care and helps build a trusting rapport with the patient.

Chief Complaint

In some EMRs, the template is selected first, and the chief complaint is delineated within the template. In other EMRs, the chief complaint is entered first, and the template stems from the chief complaint. Regardless of the format, the documentation should be accurate and complete and provide enough information to drive downstream processes. Adding a *simple free text note* can quickly provide *critical information* to subsequent providers that may not be conveyed through the sole use of the EMR click boxes.

Fast Facts

Periodically perform a self-chart review or have one of your peers do it for you. See if your documentation supports your triage decision. It is easy to "click" and move on, but we must only click on boxes that adequately represent the patient presentation and what was assessed.

Communication

Information gathered during triage can often be integrated into tracking boards in many facilities. Know which key elements are highlighted and drive treatment protocols. Become familiar with what your institution requires to be completed in triage. The following are some common essential documentation pieces:

- Arrival time
- Mode of arrival
- Chief complaint
- Associated symptoms
- Pain level
- Allergies
- Suicide screening
- Recent travel history
- Acuity level

Access to Information

Looking for a paper chart can take time and lead to delays. The use of an EMR makes data more accessible and allows for multiple care providers to retrieve and document information simultaneously. Immediate access to the past medical history, including allergies and medications from prior visits, is another benefit of using an EMR when determining a triage classification. For example, a patient presenting with a head injury and a Glasgow Coma Scale score of 15 may need to be assigned a higher acuity level than initially anticipated if the EMR shows the patient is taking warfarin, clopidogrel bisulfate, or rivaroxaban. Remember triage is a *process* designed to quickly assess patients' needs and direct care. Prioritize and focus on accessing parts of the EMR that will result in optimizing patient care outcomes. The advancement of the EMR has led to more data sharing between care providers, facilities, and pharmacies. A clear understanding of facility policies related to access of protected health information across multiple EMRs is essential as well as obtaining and documenting patient consent as indicated.

PITFALLS OF THE EMR

In the same way that the amount of detail accessed by one click in an EMR can be a positive, it can also lead to some pitfalls. Added elements and increased options to "click" can distract the provider from focusing on critical elements needed to determine a triage classification. Pitfalls include:

- Many layers to an electronic document (e.g., additional screens open with a click, which can be overwhelming)
- Nonessential screening questions that may be present in triage documents
- Too much information and cueing that may distract attention from recognizing key patient assessment signs

Fast Facts

- Familiarize yourself with facility-specific requirements for documentation during the triage process. Document as needed any additional information that helps validate decision-making processes and drive downstream practices to support high-quality care.
- Remain aware of functioning within the policy limitations of your facility and scope of practice.
- Many EMRs provide up-to-date evidence-based practice tips relating to screenings and assessments. Evaluate each one and remain alert to their applicability to each patient you triage.

(continued)

(continued)

- Pay attention to detail when you document and be careful not to make assumptions. Do not fall into the trap of "clicking" in the EMR just because it is available. Be precise!

Layout of EMR

The layout and functionality of a particular EMR can also lead to barriers in documentation. The difficulty or ease of maneuverability within the triage template can influence what is documented. If you are having difficulty accessing parts of the EMR, chances are your colleagues are as well. Communicate with your management team to make sure key elements needed for assessment are easily accessible.

Downtime and Upgrades

Technology sometimes fails, which requires backup procedures to be in place. Know what the downtime procedures are for your facility. Consider reviewing downtime processes during orientation and competency assessments. As use of the EMR increases, newer nurses will not have any experience with paper charting. Taking the time to "practice" charting on paper can minimize confusion and support ongoing high-quality care during unexpected downtimes. Patient care should continue in a smooth manner with or without the support of the EMR.

An advantage of the EMR is that upgrades can be more easily integrated into the practice setting. Know when upgrades are scheduled to occur and understand how changes may influence your practice. Be proactive in planning and continually familiarize yourself with updates in the EMR. Your patient's life may depend on it.

Fast Facts

- Think about how much or how little documentation is required to support the care decisions you have made.
- Make sure you document what you have observed, asked, or assessed.
- Nurses should maintain a heightened awareness during upgrades or downtime, as these times may affect your ability to access patient records.
- *Never let the EMR stand in the way of looking at the patient.* Turning your back to the patient while documenting on a computer can be potentially dangerous and certainly does not deliver the patient experience we should all aim to achieve. Although documentation is important, ensuring staff safety and performing a patient assessment should *always* come first.

14

Provider in Triage

Lynn Sayre Visser

> *Overcrowding in EDs is a nationwide challenge. A new focus that links hospital reimbursement to customer satisfaction adds another element to the practice of patient care. These issues have prompted creative methods of resource utilization. One solution is to place a provider (e.g., medical doctor, doctor of osteopathy, nurse practitioner, or physician assistant) in triage to mitigate overcrowding challenges; reduce wait times; and rapidly and efficiently assess, diagnose, and initiate care for patients. This chapter offers ideas related to process and teamwork initiatives as well as communication tips that can help improve the communication and productivity of triage teams and enhance collaboration.*

Upon conclusion of this chapter, you will be able to:

1. State the purpose of placing a provider in triage.
2. Discuss the importance of communication in triage.
3. List three tips for a provider in triage.

PURPOSE OF PLACING A PROVIDER IN TRIAGE

Placement of a provider in triage serves a multitude of functions and offers numerous potential benefits that influence quality of care. These benefits may include:

- Earlier completion of the medical screening exam (MSE)
- Faster initiation of a treatment plan (e.g., diagnostic tests, pain intervention)

- Improved patient flow and decreased departmental congestion
- Faster execution of patient disposition
- Decreased number of patients left without being seen (LWBS)
- Decreased patient length of stay (LOS)
- Increased patient and staff satisfaction

Some facilities have found that implementing the provider in triage during peak hours meets many of the purposes previously identified, resulting in increased revenue from a decreased LWBS rate. Additionally, the time from the patient's arrival at the facility to the time seen by a provider is a key factor in patient satisfaction. Many studies have demonstrated a reduction in this time frame, which is often referred to as the "door-to-doctor" or "door-to-provider" time metric. When benchmarking demonstrates a positive impact of placing the provider in triage, the hours the provider is present in triage can expand, further enhancing the positive impact on patient care.

ROLES OF STAFF AT TRIAGE

If implementing a provider in triage for the first time, developing roles for each of the team players can help build the foundation for the process. Recognizing that *flexibility* is pivotal to smooth operations at triage is essential. Although guidelines should be in place for staff roles in triage, these should be merely guidelines, with each team player collaborating to complete the work and meet patient needs. Roles to consider defining include:

- Triage registered nurse: When two nurses work together, define primary and secondary triage roles (e.g., rapid triage assessment nurse and comprehensive triage assessment nurse); see Chapter 6 for additional information
- Provider (e.g., medical doctor, nurse practitioner, physician assistant)
- Scribes (assist provider with documentation)
- Secretary, unlicensed personnel, or paramedic/emergency medical technician

Consider identifying who will perform the following:

- Rapid triage assessment and documentation
- Comprehensive triage assessment and documentation (completing a rapid triage assessment on all incoming patients is always the first priority)
- Provider documentation (e.g., provider or scribes)
- Order entry into computer systems
- Initiation of provider orders (e.g., give medications, draw labs)
- Documentation of patient going to and from radiology or other departments

- Follow-up on test results if patient remains in waiting room (WR)
- Reassessment if provider orders were initiated (e.g., effects of medication)
- Discharge of patients from the WR

COMMUNICATION

Communication is an integral component of teamwork and helps meet the purpose of placing a provider in triage. Limited or absent communication in the triage area could lead to duplication of procedures, missed orders, or delayed interventions, all of which create inefficient processes. Ultimately the purpose of implementing a provider in triage may fail and patient needs are not met. Have you ever gone to medicate a patient who stated, "The nurse just gave me that pill"? Or have you had a patient say, "When am I going to x-ray? I have waited an hour." And then you realize the x-ray was never ordered. These situations may occur frequently if effective communication and efficient processes are not in place.

Communication Within the Triage Team

Crucial communication within the triage team, whether provided verbally or with visual cues, should include:

- An understanding of the treatment plan by both the provider and nurse; this can be most easily accomplished when the provider and triage nurse work together in unison while interviewing and assessing the patient
- Systems that let the team know what parts of the treatment plan have been completed, for example:
  - Indicating patient location (e.g., in WR, x-ray) and procedures (e.g., labs, x-ray) completed in the electronic medical record (EMR)
  - Utilizing a color-coded flag system that indicates the patient has gone to x-ray, needs laboratory samples drawn, and so on

Fast Facts

Communication between the members of the triage team is vital because communication is the core of efficiency at triage. Without effective communication, ordering of diagnostic procedures can be missed, orders duplicated, or charts misplaced, leading to frustration for the staff and the patient.

Communication Between the Triage Nurse and Charge Nurse/Patient Flow Coordinator

Ongoing communication between the triage nurse and charge nurse or patient flow coordinator is essential to place patients most efficiently in the most appropriate treatment location within the facility and to assist with departmental flow. Effective communication allows for a smooth transition for both the patient and caregivers involved. Have you ever arranged for a high-acuity patient in triage to be taken to a room only to find that the bed is now occupied by an ambulance patient who just arrived? Suggestions for enhancing communication include:

- Maintaining an updated tracking board or EMR indicating filled/available rooms, isolation needs, etc.
- Communicating via electronic equipment (e.g., cell phones, hands-free wearable devices, alphanumeric pagers, walkie-talkies)

Communication Between Triage Staff and Other Departments

Ensure processes are in place for the triage team to communicate directly with other departments that help facilitate patient care, diagnostic testing, facility safety, and customer service. Departments that the triage team should be able to communicate directly with include:

- Security
- Laboratory
- Radiology
- Environmental services
- Trauma team
- Administration (e.g., nursing supervisor)

Suggestions for enhancing communication between these teams include:

- Computer access to visualize patient treatment needs from different departments that have a role in the patient's care (for facilities with EMR)
- Placement of a simple camera positioned toward the tracking board that can be viewed from other departments (for facilities where integrative EMR does not exist); access is only for departments pertinent to the patient's direct care (confidentiality needs to be maintained)
- Utilization of different-colored flags or stickers to indicate patients waiting for laboratory testing, radiology, and so on

Communication Between Triage Staff and Patients or Their Support Systems

A provider in triage can expedite the time frame in which diagnostic testing begins and treatment remedies are delivered. Although this increased efficiency is beneficial to the patient and departmental flow, too much of a good thing is not always good. If several diagnostic procedures (e.g., laboratory tests, x-rays) are ordered, along with medications, and these tests are initiated rapidly, one of the problems the staff may encounter is lack of communication with the patient about the plan of care. Suggestions for enhancing communication include:

- Communicating with patients that orders initiated by the provider in triage are intended to seek diagnostic answers more rapidly and expedite their ED visit
- Explaining that early initiation of tests may require the patient to move from the WR and back multiple times or require initiation of an intravenous line at a later time
- Stressing that the triage staff is doing everything possible to obtain a timely diagnosis and treatment plan and ensure the patient's medical stability
- Explaining that, if the condition warrants placement in the main ED for further treatment, additional tests may be ordered and another provider may be involved in the patient's care
- Informing the patient that he or she may need to change into a gown for further evaluation

Fast Facts

In an efficient triage system, multiple staff members may interact with patients and their support systems in a short period of time. Upon the patient's arrival, this initial interaction may include a simultaneous process involving the medical provider asking questions; the triage nurse documenting information; unlicensed personnel simultaneously obtaining vital signs, an electrocardiogram, and a weight; and registration inquiring about the spelling of the patient's name and his or her date of birth. Imagine how overwhelming this experience must feel to the patient. For some individuals the perception may be, "All these people are here. I must be dying!" Explain to the patient that these interactions are necessary to ensure the delivery of the highest quality of care. Let patients know the process they are experiencing is routine. The last thing a triage nurse wants is for every presenting patient to think the efficient triage process means something catastrophic is occurring.

KEY TIPS FOR THE PROVIDER

Working in triage may be uncomfortable for many providers. Historically the provider was located behind closed doors and could approach patients on his or her own time schedule.

However, in today's healthcare system, many providers are finding themselves as one of the first faces in the patient's access to healthcare. A few tips for the triage provider to follow:

- Be flexible and share the space with the triage staff, registration, and so on.
- Do not get caught up in the intricacies of triage and forget the little things like introducing yourself to both the patient and his or her support system; customer service *really* matters.
- Determine if the provider or nurse will drive the initial patient interview.
- Work in unison with the triage team members to efficiently obtain information.
- Recognize that the provider helps determine the patient destination (e.g., main ED, fast-track area, discharge from WR).
- Limit the physical exam to key assessments that are needed to determine initial orders:
    - Save more lengthy assessments for the medical providers in the main ED/fast-track area.
- When a written order for an oral contrast agent is received from the provider while the patient is in the WR, initiate giving the contrast material even if the CT scan is not formally ordered at triage (if your facility policies and procedures permit this); initiating contrast agent administration early will potentially provide a faster diagnosis, save the patient a lot of time, and prevent a situation in which the patient is left for hours on a gurney, waiting for the contrast material to move through the body.
- Manage expectations as well as the unexpected:
    - Let the patient know the provider in triage is a benefit, enabling his or her care to begin earlier while waiting for a treatment bed.
    - Explain that another provider may later ask similar or additional questions and another clinical assessment may be necessary at that time.
    - Explain that other patients may arrive later and go to a treatment area sooner due to differing patient acuity levels or treatment/placement needs within the facility.
- Treat and discharge simpler cases from the triage area:
    - Let patients and their family know you are doing them a service by tending to their needs quickly; in essence, your service is above and beyond what they should expect.

Despite the many needs at triage, do not forget why a provider is placed in triage. Becoming focused on the one sick patient before you is a natural tendency, but the goal of the provider in triage is to identify patients with high-risk or life-threatening circumstances and to move those patients back to the treatment area and initiate care on the remaining patients waiting. Avoid becoming engulfed in caring for one sick patient, as your role is to meet the needs of many.

Considerations for Triage

Open communication with the patient and support systems at triage is essential to setting the tone for expectations of the visit. Many patients arrive with chronic conditions that will most likely not be diagnosed or cured while in your facility. However, explaining that staff are excellent at ensuring no life-threatening condition exists can go a long way in easing the worry of the people sitting in front of you. Communicate, communicate, communicate!

DISCHARGES FROM THE WAITING ROOM

A provider in triage can often identify simple cases that can be discharged from the WR, reserving the hot commodity of an ED bed for a higher-acuity patient. The types of patients who may be treated and discharged from triage should be driven by the facility's policies and protocols. Patients to consider discharging from triage may require:

- A prescription only
- One test (e.g., x-ray, urinalysis)
- One or two treatment medications

Limiting the discharge focus to patients who need fewer resources helps maintain the flow of triage and minimizes situations in which triage personnel become bogged down with a multitude of additional tasks. The most important goals of triage must never be overlooked regardless of a provider working in the triage area. All incoming patients must continually be assessed to determine how quickly they need to be seen and how sick they appear to be. In essence, a rapid triage assessment should be performed on all incoming patients. If the triage nurse becomes engulfed in initiating provider orders, rather than focusing on assessing incoming patients, the foundation of triage will be lost.

Challenges of Discharging Patients From the WR

When patients are rapidly discharged from triage, challenges can occur that include:

- Failure to complete the registration process
- Lack of education delivered to the patient about the diagnosis
- Perception on the part of the patient that not being evaluated in a room with a gurney means he or she is being "kicked to the curb" without adequate treatment

If patients are discharged from the WR, steps must be in place to ensure all elements of the patient medical record are completed in the same manner as if the patient were in a treatment bed or area. Routine discharge paperwork and explanations should be provided and not limited by overcrowding or lack of triage personnel. If corners are cut so a patient can be discharged from triage, the facility may be doing the person a disservice. Patients may not understand their discharge instructions or potential complications of their conditions, which could ultimately put them at risk.

Benefits of Discharging From the WR

When the same high level of care is delivered at triage as would be experienced in the main treatment area, discharging a patient from the triage area or WR serves many benefits. These benefits include:

- Decreased department congestion
- Decreased patient length of stay
- Increased customer satisfaction

IMPLEMENTING A PROVIDER IN TRIAGE PROGRAM

Many challenges can occur when implementing a provider in triage process for the first time. Careful planning is essential to the success of the new system. Consider the following:

- Develop a provider in triage process improvement team that includes management, registered nurses, physicians, physician assistants, nurse practitioners, unlicensed personnel, secretaries, and ancillary staff from other departments.
- Identify system challenges.
- Define triage team roles.
- Create a plan/map that visually shows how the patient or staff will move within the system.
- Consider developing a core triage team of nurses and providers.
- Trial the system for short periods of time during low census hours.
- Identify what works and what does not.
- Consider the impact on back-end processes and create plans for improvement.
- Redefine the process.
- Implement the newly defined system and identify issues.
- Reanalyze the process as a team on an ongoing basis.
- Implement changes as needed.
- Share successes with the staff (e.g., decreased LOS and LWBS).

Even the best of systems breaks down at times. In an era of increasing patient volumes and higher-acuity levels, staff should recognize that failures are an opportunity to improve. Do not give up if the first efforts at implementing a provider in triage program seem like a catastrophe. Change is hard. Change can be slow. Rather than aborting what may feel like a failed project, go back to the drawing board, reconsider goals, and try again. Your patients will benefit immensely from successful changes in the end.

Fast Facts

- The first and foremost role of the triage nurse is to obtain a rapid triage assessment upon the patient's initial presentation to the facility. Assessing all incoming patients should always be the priority. Never let the efficient process of having a provider in triage interfere with the basics of the triage system unless the provider is also available to simultaneously evaluate the patient immediately upon arrival.
- System changes do not occur overnight but rather require careful planning and a team approach. Involving staff representatives from all levels of care and including staff from other departments is a must!

15

Advanced Triage Protocols

Dawn Friedly Gray

> *Increases in patient volumes and the need to expedite high-quality care have challenged healthcare leaders to implement creative methods in order to meet ongoing patient demands. The use of advanced triage protocols (ATPs) is one approach to working with these challenges. Understanding the purpose of ATPs and implementing them during the triage process can increase patient and staff satisfaction, decrease long wait times, and improve patient throughput while simultaneously enhancing patient safety. This chapter reviews the key concepts of ATPs and provides ideas for how to utilize ATPs to support patient care.*

Upon conclusion of this chapter, you will be able to:

1. Understand what ATPs are and why they are used.
2. State considerations and concerns about ATPs.
3. Explain common ATPs and key points to remember.

WHAT ARE ATPS, AND WHY ARE THEY USED?

The rate and rhythm of how patients arrive at a facility can vary greatly. Ensuring delivery of safe, high-quality care should be maintained at all times despite volume and acuity influxes. ATPs can direct care processes to continue regardless of routine or unexpected delays and are helpful when a medical provider or a treatment area is not immediately available.

Key Aspects of Protocols

- Unique to each facility and require administrative approval
  - This cannot be emphasized enough. Make sure you know the facility-specific protocols where you work!
- Based on the chief complaint or specific disease conditions and the triage assessment
- Include diagnostic, therapeutic, and clinical management aspects
- Provide standardized treatment guidelines
- Evidence-based

Why Use ATPs?

Initiating ATPs has many benefits. Delays in care and higher lengths of stay have been shown to occur when patients seek help for lower-acuity conditions. Current trends have facility administrators evaluating front-end measurements. One front-end measurement commonly assessed is the time from patient arrival to when a medical provider makes patient contact and care is initiated. This time frame is often referred to as the "door-to-doctor" or "door-to-provider" time. The implementation of ATPs can decrease wait times and expedite clinical decision-making. With facility policies in place, nurses can initiate diagnostic assessments to begin immediate intervention and facilitate patient care when necessary.

Early initiation of diagnostic testing, pain management therapy, fever control treatment regimens, and tetanus vaccination protocols can decrease front-end delays and increase patient satisfaction. Timely identification of abnormal treatment results leads to safer patient outcomes and high-quality care delivery. Staff satisfaction is improved by increased nurses' autonomy and enhanced interprofessional collaboration.

> **Fast Facts**
>
> - ATPs can be used to initiate care processes and expedite patient throughput while increasing patient and staff satisfaction. Consider implementing ATPs in your facility if common delays occur.

COMMON CONSIDERATIONS AND CONCERNS

Implementation of ATPs requires careful attention to the many details and processes involved for guidelines to be successful.

Initiation of Protocols

Knowing the guidelines and expectations of your facility is imperative to appropriately initiate ATPs. For example, does your facility policy support starting protocols on all patients or only when immediate bedding is not available? Protocols tend to be generalized according to a patient's complaint. Are you allowed to tweak ATPs if the chief complaint does not match a specific treatment pathway? For example, a chief complaint of abdominal pain in a 50-year-old man with a past medical history (PMH) of alcoholism may require different testing than a 50-year-old man with abdominal pain and no PMH. Also, initiation of protocols is only beneficial if adequate support staff are available to perform the ordered laboratory testing and ECGs and transport patients to radiology for x-ray, ultrasound, and other testing.

Reviewing Results

ATPs are initiated with the hope that a treatment room and provider will be available in a short amount of time. As we know, this is not always the case. There is an added responsibility on the triage nurse to review results and identify abnormal results so they may be reported to the medical provider. Upgrading or downgrading of the acuity level may be necessary, which may change the care requirements for the patient; however, *the original acuity level will not change*. Additionally, facility policies should outline actions to be taken if protocols have been initiated and the patient leaves before being seen by a provider.

Fast Facts

- When implementing ATPs, be sure to follow guidelines from facility policies, nurse practice acts, and governing agencies and organizations, including the Centers for Medicaid and Medicare Services, the Joint Commission, and the Emergency Nurses Association.
- Each nurse is responsible for knowing the limitations and regulatory requirements governing his or her licensure. Remain sensitive to using clinical judgment and do not hesitate to collaborate with medical providers when necessary.

Educational Requirements

Additional training is required for all nurses who initiate ATPs. Identification of unusual case presentations and quick assessment skills are a few of the specialized skills necessary to ensure quality outcomes in patient care. Nurses need to have experience providing care for patients of all ages with varied chief complaints to support advanced understanding and identification of subtle and clinically important differences in individual patient presentations. Utilizing

ATPs involves more than just picking a protocol to initiate care processes. Knowing what questions to ask to narrow down and pinpoint which protocol should be started is critical. Frequent reviews and ongoing assessments are essential to support best practices during triage processes.

> ### Fast Facts
>
> - Know what policies and guidelines govern the use of ATPs where you work. Stay abreast of evidence-based practices and encourage your facility's administration to make changes to standing protocols when indicated.
> - Resist becoming complacent and following rote practices when ATPs are used.
> - Your assessment skills should be patient centered and based on clinical judgment. You are the best advocate for the patient!

REVIEW OF COMMON TRIAGE PROTOCOLS

Most facilities divide ATPs into different chief complaints and patient presentations. Laboratory testing and radiology orders can vary greatly. In most states, medication administration requires a specific order and is not included in protocols. However, some facilities do include routine and time-sensitive medication administration in protocols (e.g., acetaminophen, ibuprofen, tetanus immunization, nebulizers, aspirin, and nitroglycerin). Knowing your facility's guidelines is imperative. This section provides general protocol categories and highlights some special considerations.

Abdominal Pain

- Complete metabolic panel (CMP), including amylase/lipase, complete blood count (CBC), urinalysis (UA), urine culture and sensitivity (urine C&S)
- Urine human chorionic gonadotropin (hCG) pregnancy test, quantitative serum hCG when appropriate
- Consider obtaining an ECG in patients older than 40 years of age; atypical presentations may be cardiac in origin
- Provide the patient with nothing by mouth (NPO)
- Additional testing (usually requires additional medical provider order) may include ultrasound (US) and CT

Altered Level of Consciousness

- ECG
- Keep patient NPO

- Blood glucose level
- CMP, CBC, UA, and serum toxicology
- Additional testing (usually requires additional medical provider order) may include a head CT scan

Chest Pain

- ECG may be required within 10 minutes of arrival; know your facility parameters
- ST-segment elevation myocardial infarction alerts, core measure standards (see Chapter 11)
- CMP, CBC, creatine phosphokinase (CPK), troponin; coagulation studies, including prothrombin time (PT), partial thromboplastin time (PTT), and international normalized ratio (INR); chest x-ray (CXR)
- Additional testing (usually requires additional medical provider order) may include B-type natriuretic peptide (BNP), D-dimer, or chest CT

Extremity Injury

- Be aware of individual facility standards and know what common views may be requested by the radiologist; x-rays can be tricky to order.
- Tetanus administration is often initiated with protocols; be sure to document why/why not it is administered.
- Consider initiation of a pain management protocol.

Fever

- CMP, CBC, UA, urine C&S, blood cultures (two sets), CXR
- Consider sepsis alert; additional protocols may be included in sepsis bundles, such as lactate levels and early administration of fluids and antibiotics
- Fever control protocols can be based on age, weight, or temperature and some protocols allow for alternating acetaminophen/ibuprofen administration for persistent fever in children; do not forget to reassess temperature as indicated

Neurological Symptoms

- CMP, CBC, PT, PTT/INR, and serum toxicology
- Blood glucose level
- CXR
- Dysphagia screening, NPO status
- Consider initiating a stroke alert per policy if the time of onset of symptoms is known and there is the potential for life-saving/life-enhancing intervention; refer to Chapter 11 for additional information

- Additional testing (usually requires additional medical provider order) may include head CT scan

Pain Management

- Administration of oral analgesics can be based on age and severity.
- Consider NPO status limitations and reassessment parameters.

Psychological Complaints

- CMP, CBC, urine and serum toxicology
- Evaluate the need for suicide precautions

Shortness of Breath

- CMP, CBC, CPK, troponin, PT, PTT/INR, D-dimer, and BNP
- ECG and CXR
- Additional testing (usually requires additional medical provider order) may include chest CT scan

Vaginal Bleeding

- CBC and type & Rh (rhesus), urine hCG, and quantitative serum hCG if pregnant
- Additional testing (usually requires additional medical provider order) may include pelvic US exam

> **Fast Facts**
>
> - ATPs vary greatly and should support facility goals to improve throughput and maintain high-quality care. Consider leading a facility-based effort to implement ATPs if currently not in practice. Continually evaluate protocols to expedite care and ensure best practices.

V

"Red Flag" Patient Presentations

16

Introduction to "Red Flag" Presentations

Lynn Sayre Visser

The stage for success at triage has been set. Now what? Envision the patients rolling through the doors. How will you sort through the volumes of people presenting for medical care? Who will receive the last open gurney? Determining at triage whether a patient's complaint is a high acuity level or a low acuity level can be challenging. What is important to unveil is enough information to identify those conditions that are either life-threatening or potentially life-threatening, require time-sensitive treatment, or need rapid intervention. This chapter provides a foundation for the triage process, "red flag" findings, worst-case scenarios, questions, assessments, and interventions, which should be considered for all patient presentations. The chapters that follow focus on the specifics of each body system.

Upon conclusion of this chapter, you will be able to:

1. State three worst-case scenarios for any patient presentation.
2. List three generic triage questions that apply to all patient presentations.
3. List three "red flag" findings for any presentation.

THE TRIAGE PROCESS

Regardless of the type of facility where you work, each patient seeking medical treatment deserves the same level of diligent care that you would expect for yourself. Consistent use of best practices and a systematic approach to triage should be implemented. This systematic process involves these steps:

- Across-the-room assessment
- Eliciting the chief complaint
- The patient interview
- The physical assessment (quick focused exam)
- Vital signs

Across-the-Room Assessment

The across-the-room assessment marks the beginning of triage. To adequately assess a patient upon arrival and prevent missing critical observations, visibility of the waiting room is a must. The person performing the across-the-room assessment should use all his or her senses to obtain a general overview of the patient's physiological status. Not only is information about airway, breathing, circulation, and disability obtained through observation, but sights, sounds, and smells provide a great deal of information. This initial impression may indicate the patient is a high acuity level and no additional time needs to be spent obtaining information. Treatment is the priority. Remember triage is a *process*, not a place.

Eliciting the Chief Complaint

A *licensed and qualified* member of the triage team should determine the patient's chief complaint. As discussed in Chapter 10, the patient's perceived chief complaint is *not necessarily* the actual chief complaint. Thus, careful questioning by a medical person trained to obtain the chief complaint is essential.

The Patient Interview

After a clear and concise chief complaint is obtained, the triage nurse can begin to focus on the questions, acquiring valuable information that helps determine the triage acuity level. To be most efficient, the triage nurse should drive the line of questioning using a systematic approach. Using a combination of closed and open-ended questions assists the nurse in obtaining all pertinent information.

The Physical Assessment

The triage physical assessment should be brief, structured, and driven by the chief complaint. However, the triage team must *never* become so narrowly focused that the nurse misses seeing the bigger picture. For example, if the patient has a chest complaint, investigation of both the cardiac and pulmonary systems is important and may require auscultating heart tones or lung sounds. A *visual assessment* of the area of injury or complaint is a vital component of the triage process. Patients might minimize their symptoms or not be aware of the severity of their condition. The subtle clues that become apparent during the nurse's line of questioning and physical assessment are often the answers needed to justify the acuity level. The patient may arrive complaining of a cut to the arm with a bandage in place. Initially, the nurse could think this is a low-acuity patient, but upon removing the bandage, an arterial bleed becomes evident.

Vital Signs

The degree to which vital signs are obtained at triage depends on the *urgency* of the patient's medical condition. If the across-the-room assessment provides enough information to determine a high-acuity presentation and immediate bedding criteria are met, the patient goes straight to a treatment bed *without* obtaining vital signs. Vital signs are a piece of the puzzle in triage decision-making and *may* lead the nurse to increase the patient acuity level.

Fast Facts

- The vital signs obtained upon the patient arrival serve as a baseline. Ensuring the *accuracy* of the initial set of vital signs is critical in evaluating the patient and guiding the treatment plan. The nurse obtaining the vital signs should always use critical thinking when considering if the vital signs correlate with the patient condition and assessment findings.
- Automatic vital sign machines should *never* be a substitute for correlating data by palpating pulses, counting the respiratory rate, and manually confirming an abnormal blood pressure. For example, if a pulse oximetry reading is low, the nurse should consider whether the patient presentation confirms the low reading.
- Staff should always consider whether the patient has a temperature (e.g., oral, tympanic) that correlates with the skin temperature. For example, if the patient is flushed and the face is hot to touch after obtaining a temperature within normal limits, then the nurse should consider repeating the temperature or utilizing an alternative method.

The Patient Acuity Level

The chapters that follow will not indicate the acuity level of each presentation, as many variables play a role in this decision-making. Patient presentations vary, and risk factors differ. What is important to note is that the presentations discussed are worst-case scenarios that the nurse should *consider*. When the worst-case scenario cannot be ruled out, the triage nurse will likely find the presentation to be a high acuity level based on the acuity scale criteria.

RED FLAG FINDINGS

Each chapter presents "red flag" findings that, aside from rare circumstances, are most likely high-acuity presentations. These presentations should cause the nurse to think: *Act fast!* The "red flag" findings that follow may be evident with any body system complaint. Additionally, the triage nurse should consider whether the patient is progressively worsening over time and use that information in conjunction with the clinical findings:

- Airway compromise
- Apneic
- Cardiopulmonary arrest
- Cyanotic, gray, unusually pale, diaphoretic
- Hyperthermia
- Hypothermia
- Life-threatening dysrhythmia
- New-onset confusion
- New-onset limb weakness or paralysis
- Respiratory failure or distress
- Syncopal episode with unknown etiology
- Unable to speak (abnormal for patient)
- Unresponsive

WORST-CASE SCENARIOS

Under this heading in the chapters that follow, many worst-case scenarios for the specific body system are listed in alphabetical order. The compact size of this book does not allow for every potential patient presentation or worst-case scenario to be discussed. However, the worst-case scenarios covered provide a foundation upon which the triage nurse can build. *A significant impairment to the patient's airway, breathing, circulation, or neurological status is a worst-case scenario for every patient regardless of the presenting complaint.* This point will not be repeated in each chapter but is always concerning, and it is a clinical finding that requires action.

ESSENTIAL TRIAGE QUESTIONS, ASSESSMENT, AND INTERVENTIONS

The generic questions, assessment, and interventions that follow should be *considered* for *all* patient presentations.

Generic Questions

- Reason for your visit?
- Onset and course of symptoms?
- Recent fever?
- Recent travel (e.g., another country or region)?
- Recent exposure to an infectious disease?
- Treatment prior to arrival (e.g., medication given, ice, splint, etc.)?
- Did the pain begin before the onset of symptoms?
- Pain characteristics (PQRST: provokes and palliates, quality, region and radiation, severity and associated symptoms, timing and temporal relations)?
- Associated systemic symptoms (e.g., nausea, shortness of breath, diaphoresis, feeling faint)?
- Medical, surgical, social, and family history?
- Medications and allergies?
- Immunization status?

Generic Assessment

- *Airway:* Patent or impaired (e.g., stridor, hoarseness, drooling, facial or oropharyngeal edema)
- *Breathing:* Unlabored or labored (e.g., accessory muscle use, retractions, nasal flaring)
- *Circulation:* Skin color (e.g., pallor, cyanosis) and moisture (e.g., dry, moist, diaphoretic); pulse rate (e.g., fast or slow) and rhythm (e.g., regular or irregular); obvious bleeding
- *Disability (neurological status):* Level of consciousness, including Glasgow Coma Scale (GCS) or alert, verbal, pain, unresponsive (AVPU) scale; assessing for muscle strength in upper extremities (e.g., pronator drift, grips) and lower extremities (e.g., ability to lift both legs?)
- *Exposure/Environment:* Hyperthermic, hypothermic, or normothermic; presence of objects or forensic evidence requiring preservation
- *Vital signs* (e.g., heart rate, respiratory rate, blood pressure, pulse oximetry, and pain scale)

Generic Interventions

- Intervene immediately in patients with any airway, breathing, circulation impairment, or disability and/or requiring exposure/environmental control.

- Consider the administration of oxygen per protocol or advocate accordingly.
- Document arrival time at triage and use this as "time zero" for implementing care; think core measure criteria and refer to Chapter 10 to initiate care if criteria are met (e.g., acute myocardial infarction, stroke, pneumonia).
- Consider preservation of forensic evidence if indicated.
- Consider the need to take action in patients with abnormal vital signs.
- Anticipate cooling for hyperthermia or drying and warming for hypothermia patients.
- Give nothing by mouth (NPO) if anticipating surgical intervention or conscious sedation (e.g., suspected fracture, dislocation).
- Advocate for rapid room placement; see Chapter 6 for more on immediate bedding criteria.
- Advocate for a timely diagnostic workup and initiation of care for patients with a suspicion of a high-acuity presentation.
- Consider transporting the patient to the treatment area by wheelchair or gurney.
- Consider analgesics per protocol or advocate as needed.
- Perform frequent patient reassessment per acuity scale criteria and facility protocols.

SPECIFIC CONDITIONS

In the "red flag" patient presentation chapters that follow, the specific conditions listed under this heading are arranged in alphabetical order and have other questions or assessments that may lead the nurse to rule in or rule out the potential worst-case scenario. The triage nurse *will not diagnose* the patient; rather, the information obtained helps drive the questioning and may further validate the need for assigning a high-acuity level. The information under each potential worst-case scenario is not intended to be comprehensive in nature but rather provides the triage nurse with key considerations while working through the nursing process.

Fast Facts

Each patient presenting to triage deserves a *nonjudgmental* assessment based on assimilation of information, including the triage interview, physical assessment, and vital signs. The triage team must *look* at the area(s) of complaint and consider whether all the information, including the patient's complaint, color, demeanor, and vital signs, makes clinical sense. If something seems off, further investigation should occur.

17

Respiratory Emergencies

Polly Gerber Zimmermann and Lynn Sayre Visser

Determining at triage whether a complaint is respiratory or cardiac in origin can be challenging, and more often than not, the answer may not come until after diagnostic testing. Because chest pain and shortness of breath often go hand in hand, a careful review of both the respiratory and cardiac emergency chapters can help prepare the nurse for assessing these patient populations. This chapter provides a foundation for potential high-acuity respiratory presentations that the triage nurse may encounter. See Chapter 18 for other presentations not addressed in this chapter.

Upon conclusion of this chapter, you will be able to:

1. State three worst-case scenarios of respiratory presentation.
2. List three triage questions related to a respiratory emergency.
3. List three "red flag" findings of respiratory emergencies.

RED FLAG FINDINGS

- Accessory muscle use, retractions, and/or nasal flaring
- Breath sounds unilateral or absent
- Confusion or restlessness
- Look of fear or describing a feeling of impending doom
- Respiratory distress (severe) or respiratory failure

- Shortness of breath with associated chest pain
- Speaks only one or two words or clipped sentences
- Trauma to the chest, blunt or penetrating
- Unresponsive

WORST-CASE SCENARIOS

Anaphylaxis, epiglottitis, foreign body obstruction, inhalation injury, Ludwig's angina, peritonsillar abscess, pertussis, pneumonia, pulmonary embolism, respiratory distress/respiratory failure (e.g., asthma, chronic obstructive pulmonary disease, heart failure, pulmonary edema), tension pneumothorax, tuberculosis.

ESSENTIAL TRIAGE QUESTIONS, ASSESSMENT, AND INTERVENTIONS

Chapter 16 is a crucial foundation for the content that follows.

Generic Questions

- Shortness of breath?
- Chest pain or pain with inspiration?
- What began first, the shortness of breath or the chest pain (if both present)?
- Recent fever?
- Presence of a cough (productive or nonproductive)?
- Producing sputum (e.g., color, evidence of blood, consistency)?
- Difficulty swallowing?
- Recent travel (e.g., concern for severe acute respiratory syndrome [SARS] or other diseases)?
- Known exposure to infectious disease?
- Recent upper respiratory infection?
- Smoking history?

Generic Assessment

- Respiratory rate, depth, rhythm
- Labored or unlabored respirations
- Accessory muscle use, retractions, nasal flaring
- Number of words patient is able to speak
- Facial or oropharyngeal edema
- Drooling
- Skin color
- Level of consciousness (e.g., restlessness)
- Peripheral edema
- Lung sounds

Generic Interventions

- Initiate basic life support measures.
- Institute continuous monitoring of airway for progressive airway compromise.
- Place a surgical mask on the patient if cough present.
- Initiate respiratory isolation if indicated.
- Consider initiation of oxygen per protocol or advocate accordingly.

Fast Facts

- Respiratory complaints can progress rapidly, leading to a sudden change of acuity.
- If a patient who is waiting states that breathing is becoming more difficult, the tongue feels swollen, or he or she expresses a sense of impending doom, *believe the patient* and reassess! Triage nurses should never let their guard down because often this is when a patient deteriorates and adverse outcomes occur.

SPECIFIC CONDITIONS

The questions, assessment, and interventions that follow are *not* intended to be comprehensive in nature but will help guide the triage nurse through the nursing process.

Anaphylaxis

1. *Questions:* Exposure to known or new allergen (e.g., seafood, peanuts and other nuts, insect bite or sting, iodine, latex, medication, or eggs); how many times did the exposure occur (for bites or stings)?
2. *Assessment:* Wheezing; rash with systemic involvement (e.g., low blood pressure); facial, tongue, or lip swelling; significant pruritus
3. *Intervention:* Anticipate medication orders (e.g., epinephrine, bronchodilators, antihistamines, steroids, H_2 blockers, and nebulizer treatments)

Epiglottitis

1. *Questions:* Sudden onset of symptoms; sore throat (noted in 95% of patients), odynophagia or dysphagia (noted in 95% of patients)?
2. *Assessment:* Muffled voice, inspiratory stridor (a late finding), tripod position, drooling; irritability; toxic appearance

3. *Interventions:* Limit activity and stimulation during and after assessmen; keep child with parent or caregiver and minimize stressors; place in position of comfort

Foreign Body Obstruction: Partial or Complete

1. *Question:* Evidence of choking?
2. *Assessment:* Look for the universal choking sign (patient holding the throat and appearing anxious); difficulty or inability to speak, stridor, presence of a cough (cough may indicate partial but not complete obstruction); look of fear/impending doom, cyanosis
3. *Interventions:* Initiate basic life support protocols for foreign body removal; limit any exertion the patient puts forth

Inhalation Injury

1. *Questions:* What was the exposure (e.g., smoke, chemicals); duration of the exposure?
2. *Assessment:* Presence of hoarse voice, stridor or cough; black-tinged sputum, soot around nostrils, singed nasal hairs or eyebrows, mouth burns; skin color (cherry red skin is often indicative of carbon monoxide poisoning; may be more difficult to see in dark-skinned individuals)
3. *Intervention:* Anticipate the delivery of 100% humidified oxygen rapidly

Fast Facts

- Any evidence of an inhalation injury should be enough for the triage nurse to be highly concerned. The patient should be immediately placed in a treatment bed and the medical provider notified due to the high risk for worsening airway edema and airway obstruction.
- Although the patient may have a pulse oximetry reading of 100%, the triage nurse must remain astute. Carbon monoxide binding to hemoglobin gives a false high pulse oximetry reading.

Ludwig's Angina

1. *Questions:* Recent dental infection, tooth abscess, or mouth injury?
2. *Assessment:* Swelling of floor of mouth, elevated tongue or neck swelling, drooling
3. *Intervention:* Continuous airway monitoring

Peritonsillar Abscess

1. *Questions:* Recent pharyngitis or tonsillitis?

2. *Assessment:* Unilateral tonsil swelling; unilateral neck swelling; muffled voice; older child, adolescent, or young adult; trismus (difficulty opening mouth); uvula displaced away from the area of swelling
3. *Intervention:* Anticipate the need for needle aspiration of abscess and antibiotics

Pertussis (Whooping Cough)

1. *Questions:* Severe cough (whooping sound), runny nose, fever, vomiting, or fatigue; any episodes of not breathing (apnea is noted in 67% of infants with pertussis); seizure-like activity; decreased urination or frequency of wetting diapers (Centers for Disease Control and Prevention, 2018)?
2. *Assessment:* Auscultate lung sounds; assess for signs of dehydration (e.g., absence of tearing, dry tongue/mucous membranes, and poor skin turgor)
3. *Intervention:* Initiate respiratory isolation per protocol

Pneumonia

1. *Questions:* Fever, shortness of breath, cough, or chest discomfort; fatigue, weakness, vomiting, or malaise; prolonged bed rest or recent surgery?
2. *Assessment:* Adventitious lung sounds; vital sign abnormality
3. *Interventions:* Anticipate the need for laboratory tests (e.g., complete blood count, blood cultures), chest x-ray (CXR), and antibiotics within 6 hours of arrival to facility; see Chapter 11 for additional information on pneumonia and screening for the possibility of sepsis

Pulmonary Embolism

1. *Questions:* Sudden-onset pleuritic chest pain; hemoptysis; taking birth control pills; recent surgery; any recent relative immobility (e.g., bedridden, recent travel, or recent hospitalization); pregnancy or postpartum; history of deep vein thrombosis, pulmonary embolism, or large bone fracture (also a risk for fat emboli); current or past history of cancer?
2. *Assessment:* Unilateral leg swelling after prolonged immobility; vital signs often reveal tachycardia, tachypnea, and low pulse oximetry; restlessness; nonspecific symptoms (often the case with pulmonary embolism and may mimic other conditions)
3. *Interventions:* Consider oxygen per protocol or advocate accordingly; consider rapid need for anticoagulants (e.g., thrombolytic agents) if hemodynamically unstable

Fast Facts

- The classic triad of symptoms for pulmonary embolism includes sudden-onset, sharp pleuritic chest pain (66% of the time), dyspnea, and hemoptysis. All three are present approximately 20% of the time. Most pulmonary emboli come from venous thromboembolism.
- At least one of the following risk factors is present in 90% of patients with a pulmonary embolism: immobility, heart disease, cancer, oral contraceptive pill use, pregnancy, previous deep venous thrombosis or pulmonary embolism, history of clotting disorders, recent surgery, hospitalization, travel, or hypercoagulability.

Respiratory Distress/Respiratory Failure

1. *Questions:* Sudden onset of symptoms; shortness of breath or chest pain; how long have the symptoms been present?
2. *Assessment:* Stridor, drooling, oropharyngeal edema; difficulty or inability to speak; skin color (e.g., pale or cyanotic); level of restlessness
3. *Interventions:* Initiate basic life support protocols; limit level of patient exertion

Tension Pneumothorax

1. *Questions:* Sudden-onset pleuritic chest pain, severe shortness of breath, dyspnea; blunt or penetrating trauma?
2. *Assessment:* Signs of decreasing cardiac output (e.g., hypotension, tachycardia, clammy skin, ECG changes); jugular vein distention; deviated trachea (points toward the "good lung"); decreased lung sounds on auscultation; restlessness or anxiety; muffled heart sounds
3. *Intervention:* Anticipate the need for immediate needle decompression if severe hemodynamic compromise is present (do not delay treatment for a CXR)

Tuberculosis

1. *Questions:* Recent fatigue, fever, chills, or night sweats; cough lasting several weeks; bloody sputum; recent weight loss; recent travel, incarceration, or exposure to a person with known tuberculosis?
2. *Assessment:* Refer to Generic Assessment discussed earlier
3. *Interventions:* Place a surgical mask on the patient; initiate airborne precautions (e.g., negative pressure room); communicate with other personnel per policy regarding isolation status

Fast Facts

- One role of the triage nurse is to limit the spread of infections to staff, patients, and visitors. During flu season and when patients or visitors are coughing, masks and tissues should be handed out judiciously to reduce the spread of germs. The more frequently masks are distributed, the less uncomfortable individuals wearing them will feel.
- If in doubt about the seriousness of a potentially communicable respiratory disease, *isolate, isolate, isolate!*

Reference

Centers for Disease Control and Prevention. (2018). Transmission of measles. Retrieved from https://www.cdc.gov/measles/about/transmission.html

18

Cardiac Emergencies

Polly Gerber Zimmermann

*Chest pain can originate from many sources and may range from acute myocardial infarction to benign costochondritis. The key responsibility at triage is to consider the worst-case scenario in determining proper priorities. In cardiac conditions, **time is muscle**. Therefore, rapid intervention for suspicious cardiac conditions is imperative. See Chapter 11 for a further understanding of timelines related to ECGs, thrombolytic therapy, and percutaneous coronary intervention. This chapter provides a foundation for potential high-risk cardiac presentations that the triage nurse may encounter.*

Upon conclusion of this chapter, you will be able to:

1. State three worst-case scenarios of cardiac presentation.
2. List three triage questions related to a cardiac emergency.
3. List three "red flag" findings of cardiac emergencies.

RED FLAG FINDINGS

- Angina different from the patient's usual characteristics
- Appears acutely ill, cyanotic/pale, clammy/diaphoretic, and/or significantly uncomfortable
- Cocaine or crack use with chest pain
- Level of consciousness altered from baseline (e.g., confusion, lethargy, or restlessness)

- Life-threatening arrhythmia
- Look of fear or feeling of impending doom
- Repetitive shocks by an implantable cardioverter defibrillator (ICD) or more than three shocks in a 24-hour period
- Sudden-onset, severe chest pain
- Syncopal episode associated with chest pain or shortness of breath
- Tracheal deviation
- Trauma to the chest, blunt or penetrating (see Chapter 27)

WORST-CASE SCENARIOS

Acute coronary syndrome (ACS), aortic dissection, endocarditis, pericardial tamponade, pericarditis

ESSENTIAL TRIAGE QUESTIONS, ASSESSMENT, AND INTERVENTIONS

Chapter 16 is a crucial foundation for the content that follows.

Generic Questions

- Chest pain or pain with inspiration?
- Syncopal episode?
- Shortness of breath?
- What began first, the chest pain or shortness of breath (if both present)?
- Sudden onset of bilateral ankle edema?
- Associated systemic symptoms (e.g., nausea, shortness of breath, diaphoresis, feeling faint)?
- Rash? (Rule out herpes zoster.)
- Recent trauma?
- History of recent upper respiratory infection (costochondritis)?
- Patient's perception of effort required to maintain oxygenation?
- Past history of similar symptoms; how is this different than previous chest pain?
- Heart disease, smoking, high blood pressure, high cholesterol, diabetes, or obesity?

Fast Facts

A patient with a recent history of forceful emesis, chest pain, and subcutaneous emphysema should raise suspicion for the triage nurse to consider Boerhaave's syndrome (e.g., tear in the esophagus).

Generic Assessment

- Respiratory rate and characteristics (normal respiration is easy and quiet)
- Ability to speak sentences, phrases, or limited number of words between breaths
- Auscultate lung sounds
- Trachea (midline or deviated)
- Altered circulation: pale, cyanotic, delayed capillary refill
- Level of consciousness (e.g., new-onset restlessness or confusion may indicate early signs of hypoxia)
- Musculoskeletal pain (usually localized, sharp, reproducible; movement makes it worse)
- Pulse oximetry (95%–100% in a healthy adult; concern is warranted if <93% without chronic illness)

Generic Interventions

- Anticipate the need for ECG within 10 minutes of arrival and continuous monitoring.
- Consider the need for oxygen for concerning chest pain, shortness of breath, or low oxygen saturation levels.

SPECIFIC CONDITIONS

The questions, assessment, and interventions that follow are *not* intended to be comprehensive in nature but will help guide the triage nurse through the nursing process.

Acute Coronary Syndrome

1. *Questions:* Discomfort of burning, pressing, or dull ache or tightness (rather than pain) to chest, jaw, neck, epigastrium, arm, or back; symptoms with exertion but relieved by rest; pain severe enough to awaken from sleep; history of hypertension, diabetes mellitus, smoking, family history of ACS, or hypercholesteremia; previous cardiac disease, coronary interventions, pacemaker, or ICD; recent use of medications for erectile dysfunction (these patients should not receive nitroglycerin); recent or past use of recreational drug use such as cocaine (can cause coronary vasospasms and accelerate coronary artery disease)?
2. *Assessment:* Altered circulation: pale, diaphoretic, cyanotic, delayed capillary refill
3. *Interventions:* Obtain an ECG within 10 minutes (refer to your facility protocol); anticipate the need for non-enteric-coated aspirin per protocol; anticipate orders for stat oxygen, ECG, intravenous access, chest x-ray (CXR), medications, and lab work

Fast Facts

- Up to 50% of patients with ACS may not have any known risk factors. ACS is classified into unstable angina, non-ST-segment elevation myocardial infarction (non-STEMI), and STEMI. Signs or symptoms of cardiac ischemia, resulting in a change in the cardiac output and perfusion, or inadequate oxygenation are a concern. *Time is muscle!* After 20 minutes of ischemia, injury begins, followed by infarction (death) within 6 to 8 hours.
- Initial negative results for an ECG or cardiac enzymes are *not* definitive. Positive results for enzymes or ECG changes are typically not seen until infarction (not ischemia) occurs. Up to 6.4% of all patients with acute myocardial infarction (AMI) had one normal ECG.
- Relief by nitroglycerin or "GI cocktail" is *not* legitimate as a diagnostic measure.
- Reproducible pain with pressure (classic in costochondritis) is *not* an absolute diagnostic measure. Up to 7% of patients with AMI or unstable angina have their pain partially or fully reproduced on chest wall palpation.

Aortic Dissection: Thoracic or Abdominal

1. *Questions:* Positional pain (usually not positional and the duration of pain lasts only hours); discomfort reveals ripping, tearing, abrupt pain, excruciating pain radiating to the anterior chest, back, abdomen, and/or lower extremities; history of hypertension, peripheral vascular disease, Marfan syndrome, or age ≥40 years?
2. *Assessment:* Check for significant differences in blood pressure and pulses between upper extremities, neurological deficits (e.g., paresthesia); auscultate for a heart murmur
3. *Interventions:* Consider oxygen per protocol; CXR stat to look for widened mediastinum

Fast Facts

- Discoloration of extremities due to poor perfusion can be indicative of aortic dissection.
- Patients with collagen vascular disorders such as Marfan syndrome are at a high risk for aortic aneurysm or dissection or both.

Endocarditis

1. *Questions:* Chest pain; joint or muscle aches; chills, fatigue, or fever; exertional shortness of breath; history of rheumatic fever or endocarditis; congenital heart abnormalities; mechanical heart valve; recent dental surgery; intravenous drug use?
2. *Assessment:* Fever; sweating; swelling of feet, legs, and/or abdomen; heart murmur
3. *Interventions:* Anticipate the need for an ECG, lab work, including two sets of blood cultures, echocardiogram, and antibiotics

Pericardial Tamponade

1. *Questions:* Sharp, stabbing pain often radiating to the shoulder, neck, back, and/or abdomen; pain worsened by deep breathing or coughing; recent open heart surgery?
2. *Assessment:* Muffled heart sounds, jugular vein distention, hypotension, or signs of shock
3. *Interventions:* Anticipate the need for immediate pericardiocentesis

Pericarditis

1. *Questions:* Sharp, sudden pleuritic chest pain that improves in upright, forward-leaning position; recent history of viral symptoms?
2. *Assessment:* Listen for pericardial rub (present in up to 69%)
3. *Intervention:* Anticipate the need for an ECG (up to 94% have abnormalities)

19

Neurological Emergencies

Reneé Semonin Holleran

There are many causes of loss of neurological function. Failure to identify concerning neurological symptoms at triage may lead to long-term disability from devastating conditions such as stroke. The history surrounding the onset of symptoms plays an important role in the care of the patient. See Chapter 11 for a further understanding of timelines of treating acute neurological conditions. This chapter provides a foundation for potential high-acuity neurological presentations that the triage nurse may encounter.

Upon conclusion of this chapter, you will be able to:

1. State three neurological presentations that are considered worst-case scenarios.
2. List three triage questions related to a neurological emergency.
3. List three "red flag" findings of neurological emergencies.

RED FLAG FINDINGS

- Change in mental status from baseline
- Difficulty breathing
- Fall(s) in a patient who uses anticoagulants
- Fever with neck stiffness
- Fever with the presence of a rash (e.g., suspicion of meningitis)
- History of ingestion of a substance that may induce neurological changes

- Inability to protect the airway
- Neurological deficits (e.g., facial droop, loss of limb function)
- Seizure (new-onset or status epilepticus)
- Worst headache of patient's life

WORST-CASE SCENARIOS

Encephalitis/meningitis, Guillain–Barré syndrome, seizure (new-onset or status epilepticus), stroke (ischemic vs. hemorrhagic)

ESSENTIAL TRIAGE QUESTIONS, ASSESSMENT, AND INTERVENTIONS

Chapter 16 is a crucial foundation for the content that follows.

Generic Questions

- Onset (time) of symptoms or injury (e.g., sudden or gradual)?
- Any injury associated with the onset of symptoms (e.g., fall before or after symptoms)?
- Pain characteristics; did the pain precede the symptoms (e.g., a severe headache before loss of function of an extremity or muscle weakness)?
- Presence of a fever or hypothermia?
  - History of ingestion of substances before changes in mental status or onset of seizure (e.g., opioids, anticoagulants, aspirin, acetaminophen)
  - History of anticoagulant use (e.g., warfarin, rivaroxaban, apixaban, etc.)
- Past medical history including diabetes (neurological changes may be related to hypoglycemia), hypertension, recent injuries, medications, and vaccination history?

Generic Assessment

- Characteristics of symptoms
  - Loss of function or weakness of an extremity
    - Sensory loss
    - Asymmetry of the face
    - Altered mental status or loss of consciousness
  - Numbness or tingling in an extremity or in the face
    - Aphasia or dysarthria
    - Dizziness
    - Increased falls
    - Urinary or bowel incontinence
- Presence of a fever or hypothermia

Generic Interventions

- Document time of witnessed changes and use this time as "time zero" for implementing care (stroke); for example, when was the patient last seen as "normal"?
- Check glucose per protocol (determine if hypoglycemia is contributing to the neurological symptoms).
  - Review the patient's current medications as possible for use of opioids or history of opioid use (administration of naloxone may change symptoms).
- Check ECG per protocol (atrial fibrillation may be the cause of stroke).

Fast Facts

When a patient presents with symptoms of stroke or other neurological changes, knowing the exact time the patient was *last seen normal* is critical information in determining the best treatment plan. "Last seen normal" refers to the patient's baseline condition.

SPECIFIC CONDITIONS

The questions, assessment, and interventions that follow are *not* intended to be comprehensive in nature but will help guide the triage nurse through the nursing process.

Encephalitis/Meningitis

1. *Questions:* Severe headache; when did it start; presence of fever or recent illness, vomiting, stiff neck, generalized weakness, or a rash noticed by patient or family?
2. *Assessment:* Change in level of consciousness (e.g., confusion); focal neurological signs, muscle weakness; fever and chills, presence of purpura or petechiae (nonblanching), nuchal rigidity
3. *Interventions:* If infection is suspected, don masks and gloves before performing patient care; isolate the patient per protocol as soon as possible, manage airway, and provide oxygen as indicated

Fast Facts

- Infants with meningitis may have a high-pitched meningeal cry and are often inconsolable. Be alert to decreased level of consciousness, poor feeding, vomiting, and/or bulging fontanelle.

(continued)

(*continued*)

- A neonate seizure can be overlooked due to its subtle symptoms (e.g., repetitive lip smacking, horizontal eye deviation, eyelid fluttering, pedaling or swimming motion). *Do not be fooled!*

Guillain–Barré Syndrome

1. *Questions:* Any history of recent upper respiratory infection; recent vaccination; any prickling, tingling sensation or weakness in lower extremities spreading upward; ascending paralysis; difficulty walking or inability to walk; difficulty swallowing or respiratory difficulties (late finding)?
2. *Assessment:* Muscle weakness; abnormal breathing patterns (late finding)
3. *Intervention:* Manage abnormal breathing patterns; patient may require bag-valve mask assistance until definitive airway management can be initiated

Seizure

1. *Questions:* History of seizure activity, tongue biting, or incontinence; what type of seizures (e.g., partial or generalized, tonic, clonic); medical history such as diabetes (hypoglycemia is potentially the cause of the seizure); postictal state; medications taken for seizures (ascertain if the patient is compliant); intentional or accidental overdose of medication; history of recent trauma or trauma due to the seizure; exposure to any toxins?
2. *Assessment:* Altered mental status; abnormal limb movement or absence of movement; bowel or bladder incontinence
3. *Interventions:* If the patient is actively seizing and there is a history of trauma, place in rescue position with cervical spine precautions; monitor airway and breathing; reposition airway as needed to remove obstruction; apply suction if needed to clear airway when possible; apply oxygen by mask if indicated

Fast Facts

- Question the patient about a history of coronary artery disease or sudden cardiac death when assessing for seizures.
- Not all tonic/clonic activity is a "seizure"; you must also consider a dysrhythmia, such as ventricular fibrillation or syncope.

Stroke (Ischemic vs. Hemorrhagic)

1. *Questions:* Onset of symptoms (*exact time*); have symptoms improved or worsened; dizziness or headache; any risk factors for stroke (e.g., hypertension, atrial fibrillation); history of trauma (e.g., a fall); recent or current use of anticoagulation medication?
2. *Assessment:* Assess stroke symptoms using a prehospital stroke assessment scale (e.g., Cincinnati Prehospital Stroke Scale); presence of facial droop, arm drift, or slurred speech
3. *Interventions:* Determine the onset of patient symptoms (administration of recombinant tissue plasminogen activator [r-tPA] needs to occur within 4.5 hours of the onset of symptoms in a patient with ischemic stroke for best outcomes); facilitate immediate medical treatment (e.g., ED)

20

Abdominal Emergencies

Polly Gerber Zimmermann and Lynn Sayre Visser

The abdomen contains many organs, both solid and hollow, that can manifest a wide range of possible abnormal findings. Utilizing key questions helps differentiate the patient with "gas" from one with a life-threatening perforation. When triaging patients, it is important to consider the worst-case scenarios and to identify not only patients who are obviously seriously ill but also those who might be. This chapter provides a foundation for potential high-acuity abdominal presentations that the triage nurse may encounter. See Chapter 21 for other presentations not addressed in this chapter.

Upon conclusion of this chapter, you will be able to:

1. State three worst-case scenarios of an abdominal presentation.
2. List three triage questions related to an abdominal emergency.
3. List three "red flag" findings of abdominal emergencies.

RED FLAG FINDINGS

- Bloody or black stools
- Boardlike or rigid abdomen (from muscle contraction)
- Coffee-ground or bloody emesis
- Acute colicky pain
- Pain severe in nature that awakens a person from sleep
- Pulsating abdominal mass
- Rebound tenderness present

- Shoulder tip pain accompanied by abdominal pain (indicates free air from perforation rising and irritating the phrenic nerve)
- Sudden-onset, severe abdominal pain

WORST-CASE SCENARIOS

Abdominal aortic aneurysm, appendicitis, cholecystitis or cholelithiasis, diverticulitis, gastrointestinal (GI) bleeding (upper and lower), esophageal varices, incarcerated hernia, intestinal obstruction (large and small intestine), pancreatitis, penile fracture, peptic ulcer disease, priapism, testicular torsion, trauma (e.g. lacerated liver, perforated intestine, splenic rupture; see Chapter 27).

ESSENTIAL TRIAGE QUESTIONS, ASSESSMENT, AND INTERVENTIONS

Chapter 16 is a crucial foundation for the content that follows.

Generic Questions

- Time of onset (acute versus gradual)?
- Vomiting (often seen in infectious processes)?
- Frequency and characteristics (e.g., color, food contents, bile appearance) of vomiting?
- Is anyone else sick in the household? Anyone sick who ate the same food?
- Emesis related to pain?
  - Pain preceding vomiting suggests a potential surgical abdomen, whereas vomiting before pain is more typical of a nonsurgical condition.
  - Nausea and vomiting occurring simultaneously with the onset of pain is associated with torsion, ectopic pregnancy, ureteral colic, or bowel obstruction.
  - Epigastric pain relieved by vomiting is more likely to be caused by an intragastric problem.
- Last bowel movement (BM)?
  - Frequency of BMs, characteristics, and normal patterns for patient?
  - Presence of dark tarry or bloody stool?
  - Guidelines for "frequent" diarrhea includes occurrence every 30 to 60 minutes for more than 6 hours, five or more episodes in the previous 24 hours, or diarrhea daily for more than 5 days.
- Passing flatus?
- Recent travel (e.g., different country or region)?
- Urine frequency (especially with children or elderly who are more prone to dehydration) and characteristics (e.g., color, odor)?

- First day of last menstrual period (if premenopausal)?
- Pain worse with movement?
- Positional pain?
  - Patients often appear rigid when flat and, if ambulating, walk gingerly to avoid moving peritoneal area; this is often referred to as the pelvic inflammatory disease (PID) shuffle.
- Previous history of the same or similar condition; does this feel the same as it did before?
- Lower chest trauma? (Remember: The liver and spleen are protected by the lower rib cage but are still vulnerable to injury.)
- Recent hospitalization, surgery, and antibiotics (within 8 weeks) with foul "horse barn odor"?
  - Rule out *Clostridium difficile* (C-Diff).

Fast Facts

- Remember that the bismuth from Pepto-Bismol and ferrous sulfate (iron) turn stools black. Stool with "digested" blood is stickier and has a foul odor.
- Atypical presentations can be "typical" in the older adult patient. Do not make assumptions regarding the origin of pain. Consider an atypical cardiac presentation in the older adult patient presenting with upper abdominal pain or nausea and vomiting. Look for the subtle clues. Approximately one third of patients older than 65 who are admitted with abdominal pain need surgery.

Generic Assessment

Vital Signs

- Abdominal pain with abnormal vital signs is usually more serious.
- Signs of dehydration
  - Heart rate is more sensitive than blood pressure (healthy adults must lose 1,500 mL of fluid before exhibiting hypotension).
  - A pulse of 120 bpm or higher is highly indicative of dehydration or other serious illness; tachycardia is an early sign.

Skin Assessment

- Assess skin turgor on sternum or forehead where alteration in skin elasticity is less marked with aging.

Abdominal Assessment

- Palpate the abdomen (consider peritoneal signs).

- Assess bowel sounds; initially bowel sounds can be hyperactive before the presence of hypoactive bowel sounds or the absence of bowel sounds with an obstruction.

Generic Interventions

- Anticipate the need for analgesics since early pain relief in stable patients with nontraumatic acute abdominal pain is recommended.
- Anticipate the need to collect urine in premenopausal women and in menstruating preadolescents/adolescents for pregnancy testing even if the patients state they are not pregnant or sexually active.
- Consider whether an ECG within 10 minutes is indicated, especially for patients with diabetes.

Fast Facts

- Severe pain that is a 7 or greater on a 0-to-10 scale and lasts 6 or more hours is a potentially serious condition.
- Writhing or restlessness is often indicative of a colicky pain from stones.
- In the older adult patient, pain out of proportion to the exam should raise concern for the potentially life-threatening diagnosis of mesenteric ischemia.
- "Frequent" vomiting is considered to be 10 or more episodes in the previous 24 hours.
- An early sign of dehydration is a decreased ability to focus.
- Areas of the body to assess for dehydration include mucous membranes, tongue, or teeth (dry). Skin can be assessed for poor turgor.

SPECIFIC CONDITIONS

The questions, assessment, and interventions that follow are *not* intended to be comprehensive in nature but will help guide the triage nurse through the nursing process.

Abdominal Aortic Aneurysm

1. *Questions:* Abdominal or back pain, or both; sudden, severe tearing pain with radiation to groin; syncopal episode; male, history of smoking, or high blood pressure (increased risk)?
2. *Assessment:* Palpate abdomen for pulsating abdominal mass or rigidity; clammy skin
3. *Intervention:* Anticipate the need for rapid surgical intervention

Appendicitis

1. *Questions:* Pain starts around umbilicus and slowly moves to right lower quadrant (McBurney's point) over 48 hours?
2. *Assessment:* Anorexia; gait with limp; rebound tenderness with abdominal assessment; age considerations (most commonly occurs in those aged 11–35 years)
3. *Intervention:* Anticipate the need for surgical intervention

Fast Facts

Patients with acute appendicitis may experience delays in diagnosis or a missed diagnosis often due to vague initial symptoms, including periumbilical and epigastric pain preceding right lower quadrant pain. Appendicitis does not only occur on the right side. The triage nurse should be aware that left-sided appendicitis may occur in patients who have an elongated appendix, situs inversus, or congenital midgut malrotation (Yang, Liu, Lin, & Lin, 2012). In pediatrics, atypical is typical.

Cholecystitis or Cholelithiasis

1. *Questions:* Time of last meal; history of recent fat intake; history of cholelithiasis; shoulder tip and acute colicky pain; presence of the six Fs (fat, female, forty, fertile, fair, flatulent)?
2. *Assessment:* Refer to Generic Assessment discussed earlier
3. *Interventions:* Give nothing by mouth (NPO) and anticipate the need for antiemetics

Diverticulitis

1. *Questions:* Constant persistent pain (sometimes for several days); nausea, vomiting, and/or constipation; fever?
2. *Assessment:* Abdominal assessment reveals left-sided pain similar to an "appendicitis"; age considerations (symptoms typically after age 50 years)
3. *Interventions:* Refer to Generic Interventions discussed earlier in this chapter

Esophageal Varices

1. *Questions:* History of cirrhosis of the liver, thrombus, or infection?
2. *Assessment:* Vomiting bright red blood; dark, tarry stools; signs of chronic liver disease (main cause); ascites; palmar erythema; spider nevi; hypovolemic shock

3. *Intervention:* Anticipate the need for oxygen, two large bore IVs, labs (e.g. CBC including type and crossmatch), possible blood transfusion; prevent vomiting (no blind nasogastric tube insertion); emergent endoscopy

GI Bleeding (Lower)

1. *Questions:* History of GI bleed (upper gastrointestinal [UGI] is more common than lower gastrointestinal [LGI]), melena? Perirectal disease, diverticulosis, cancer, or inflammatory disease (most common sources of LGI bleed)?
2. *Assessment:* Refer to Generic Assessment discussed earlier in this chapter
3. *Interventions:* Anticipate the need for nasogastric (NG) tube, labs including hemoglobin (Hgb)/hematocrit (Hct), type and crossmatch, intravenous (IV) with fluids, possible blood transfusion

GI Bleeding (Upper)

1. *Questions:* Abdominal pain? GI bleed in the last 48 to 72 hours? Dizziness or syncope? History of alcoholism or nonsteroidal antiinflammatory drug (NSAID) use? Hematemesis? History of duodenal or gastric ulcers, Mallory-Weiss tears, or esophagitis?
2. *Assessment:* Confusion, ascites, jaundice; nausea/vomiting, melena, and/or hematochezia; hypovolemia
3. *Interventions:* Refer to Generic Interventions discussed earlier in this chapter; anticipate the need for fluid replacement, labs including Hct/Hgb, type and crossmatch, blood products, endoscopy team, potential surgical intervention

Fast Facts

The volume of hematemesis is a poor guide for estimating volume loss. Tachycardia is an earlier sign followed by hypotension after 1,500 mL blood loss.

Incarcerated Hernia

1. *Questions:* History of intermittent "abdominal mass"; sudden pain with rapid increase in intensity; pain with bending over, lifting, and/or coughing?
2. *Assessment:* Palpate abdomen for "mass" that is now tender and tense
3. *Intervention:* Anticipate the need for surgical intervention

Intestinal Obstruction (Large Intestine)

1. *Question:* Obstipation (feels the need to pass gas but is unable)?
2. *Assessment:* High-pitched "tinkling" bowel sounds
3. *Interventions:* Refer to Generic Interventions discussed earlier in this chapter

Intestinal Obstruction (Small Intestine)

1. *Questions:* Vomiting (gastric contents, then bilious, then brown fecal material); symptoms worse after eating; history of abdominal surgery (present in 50%–70% of patients)?
2. *Assessment:* Refer to Generic Assessment discussed earlier in this chapter
3. *Interventions:* Refer to Generic Interventions discussed earlier in this chapter

Pancreatitis

1. *Questions:* History of alcoholism, cholelithiasis, or trauma; sudden knifelike pain in left upper quadrant, midgastric, or back (related to retroperitoneal location); is the pain worse with eating or lying flat?
2. *Assessment:* Check pulse oximetry (latent hypoxia is a major complication); signs of dehydration; hypovolemia (major complication)
3. *Intervention:* Anticipate the need for antiemetics and pain control

Penile Fracture

1. *Questions:* Activity when pain began (typically during aggressive sexual intercourse or masturbation but may include a fall or direct trauma); hear a popping sound followed by pain and loss of the erection?
2. *Assessment:* Pain, edema, discoloration (ecchymosis); blood at the meatus; hematuria or difficulty urinating
3. *Interventions:* Give nothing by mouth; anticipate the need for labs (UA to check for hematuria), pain management measures (e.g. ice), emergency urology consult and early surgical intervention to prevent erectile dysfunction or impotence

Peptic Ulcer Disease

1. *Questions:* Smoking history; generous use of NSAIDs or acetylsalicylic acid (ASA); gnawing or burning sensation intermittently?
2. *Assessment:* Vomitus for presence of blood (red or coffee-ground hematemesis); age (more common in older adults)
3. *Interventions:* Refer to Generic Interventions discussed earlier in this chapter

> **Fast Facts**
>
> Patients with duodenal ulcers have reduced pain after eating while those with gastric ulcers tend to have more pain following a meal.

Priapism

1. *Questions:* Duration of erection; difficulty urinating; history of a spinal cord injury, multiple sclerosis, stroke, sickle cell crisis, use of sexual dysfunction or psychotropic medications, or prolonged sexual activity?
2. *Assessment:* Penile engorgement or discoloration; bladder distention; increasing pain over time
3. *Interventions:* Anticipate the need to treat underlying cause (e.g. sickle cell crisis); consider ice pack and other pain management measures, as well as a urinary catheter for bladder distention; anticipate the need for nerve block injections or possible surgery

Testicular Torsion

1. *Question:* Sudden pain (often described as "twisting" after sports activities)?
2. *Assessment:* "Saddle" (bow-leg) walk; unilateral, affected testis is usually firm, and tender; intense pain or minimal pain relief when the testicle is elevated; age considerations (most common in adolescent years)
3. *Intervention:* Anticipate the need for surgical intervention

Reference

Yang, C.-Y., Liu, H.-Y., Lin, H.-L., & Lin, J.-N. (2012). Left-sided acute appendicitis: A pitfall in the emergency department. *Journal of Emergency Medicine, 43*(6), 980–982. doi:10.1016/j.jemermed.2010.11.056

21

Obstetric and Gynecological Emergencies

Lynn Sayre Visser and Polly Gerber Zimmermann

Patients seek care at triage for a variety of obstetric and gynecological presentations. Considering the worst-case scenarios and identifying not only those who are obviously seriously ill but those who might be is of utmost importance. The triage interventions for these potentially emergent presentations may be limited. However, knowledge and recognition of "red flag" findings help the nurse advocate for the patient and potentially save the life of the woman and her unborn baby. This chapter provides a foundation for potential high-acuity obstetric and gynecologic presentations that the triage nurse may encounter. See Chapter 20 for other presentations not addressed in this chapter.

Upon conclusion of this chapter, you will be able to:

1. State three worst-case scenarios of obstetric and gynecological presentation.
2. List three triage questions related to an obstetric and gynecological emergency.
3. List three "red flag" findings of obstetric and gynecological emergencies.

RED FLAG FINDINGS

- Abdominal pain in early pregnancy
- Altered mental status, headache, visual disturbances, dizziness (edema in brain)
- Amniotic fluid leaking (suspected)
- Fetal heart tones abnormally high or low
- Fetal movement absent or diminished
- Imminent delivery (perineum bulge, mother with desire to push or bear down)
- Patient states "I was sexually assaulted" or "I was raped"
- Pregnant with vaginal bleeding or passing large clots
- Protruding umbilical cord
- Seizures with known pregnancy
- Trauma in a pregnancy of greater than 24 weeks' gestation

WORST-CASE SCENARIOS

Obstetric Specific: Abruptio placentae, amniotic fluid leaking/ruptured membrane, eclampsia, ectopic pregnancy, imminent delivery, placenta previa, preeclampsia/HELLP (hemolysis, elevated liver enzyme levels, and low platelet levels) syndrome, prolapsed cord, trauma (see Chapter 27), uterine rupture

Gynecological Specific: Ovarian torsion, sexual assault, toxic shock syndrome

ESSENTIAL TRIAGE QUESTIONS, ASSESSMENT, AND INTERVENTIONS

Chapter 16 is a crucial foundation for the content that follows.

Generic Questions

- Abdominal pain or back pain? Where is the pain located (ask PQRST questions)?
- Fever?
- Nausea, vomiting, or diarrhea?
- Vaginal bleeding (quantity of tampons/pads using) or vaginal discharge (foul smelling, color)?
- Urinary tract infection signs or symptoms (e.g., increased urinary frequency, sense of urgency, dysuria)?
- First day of your last *normal* menstrual cycle?
- Any chance you may be pregnant? (The answer no does not mean the patient is not pregnant; consider that the patient *could be* pregnant yet unaware.)
- If pregnant, how many times have you been pregnant (gravida)? How many deliveries have you had (para)? Abortions? Number of babies

expecting? Estimated date of delivery? Has your water broken? Any recent medication or drug use? Receiving prenatal care?
- Uterine irritability? Rhythmic contractions? If so, how frequent are the contractions and how long do they last?
- History of known obstetric/gynecological problems currently or in the past?

Generic Assessment

- Palpate the abdomen
- Vital signs of the mother and, if pregnant, assess fetal health by fetal heart tones after the 12th week (110–160 bpm is an expected normal range)
- Fetal movement after 18 weeks (ask when the mother last felt movement; any change in fetal movement from normal)

Generic Interventions

- Consider analgesics per protocol since early pain relief in stable patients with nontraumatic acute abdominal pain is recommended (careful consideration needs to be taken with known pregnancy).
- Collect urine specimen for urinalysis per protocol or advocate accordingly.
- Collect urine for pregnancy test per protocol in female patients of childbearing age.

Fast Facts

Do not assume a person is not pregnant solely because she says she is not pregnant. At times a person may be in denial about the possibility of a pregnancy. Pregnancy must be ruled out in women with abdominal pain who are of childbearing age.

SPECIFIC CONDITIONS—OBSTETRIC RELATED

The questions, assessment, and interventions that follow are *not* intended to be comprehensive in nature but will help guide the triage nurse through the nursing process.

Abruptio Placentae

1. *Questions:* Sudden, severe abdominal pain or cramping/contractions; vaginal bleeding (expect dark-red blood); history of trauma, hypertension, or drug use (methamphetamine or cocaine)?
2. *Assessment:* Palpate abdomen (expect hard abdomen); fetal heart tones (expect abnormal fetal response)

3. *Interventions:* Transfer to treatment bed and position patient on her left side; consider the need for oxygen and anticipate preparation for possible cesarean section

Amniotic Fluid Leaking/Ruptured Membrane

1. *Questions:* Presence of any urinary tract symptoms (e.g., dysuria, hematuria, increased urinary frequency); did you feel a trickle of fluid while standing or a gush of fluid when lying down?
2. *Assessment:* Determine if fluid is urine or amniotic fluid; amniotic fluid is odorless and colorless; fetal heart tones
3. *Interventions:* Anticipate the need to perform the fern and nitrazine (pH) tests, or see if fluid gushes after lying down; if the pH is greater than 6.5, the membranes have likely ruptured

Eclampsia

1. *Questions:* How long did the seizure-like activity last, what did the seizure-like activity look like, any associated injuries, estimated due date (more than 20 weeks pregnant is high risk), recent delivery; headache, visual changes?
2. *Assessment:* Examine areas of injury; presence of tongue laceration or broken teeth; hyperreflexia; fetal heart tones (do not delay initiation of treatment to obtain fetal heart tones)
3. *Interventions:* Immediate placement in a treatment room, provide emotional support; initiate seizure precautions and protect from self-harm; anticipate the need to protect airway if patient seizes, and prepare for emergency delivery and possible magnesium sulfate infusion

Ectopic Pregnancy

1. *Questions:* Syncopal episode; missed or irregular period; minimal or absent vaginal bleeding; shoulder pain (Kehr's sign) with ruptured ectopic pregnancy; history of pelvic inflammatory disease (noted in 50% of women with ectopic pregnancies); sharp unilateral lower abdominal pain that is moderate to severe and occurs around the sixth week of gestation?
2. *Assessment:* Evidence of shock following a ruptured fallopian tube
3. *Interventions:* Anticipate the need for a human chorionic gonadotropin (hCG) blood test and expect a positive pregnancy result; foresee the need for surgical intervention

Imminent Delivery

1. *Questions:* Feel the need to bear down or push with or between contractions?
2. *Assessment:* Bulging membranes visible at vulva or crowning of the fetal head; mother states the "baby is coming" or that she is going to defecate

3. *Interventions:* Call for help; apply gentle pressure on the crown to prevent rapid expulsion (support perineum to reduce tearing); allow head to rotate naturally; feel for the umbilical cord around the neonate's neck and unwrap if necessary once head is delivered; deliver the shoulders by guiding head downward (to deliver the anterior shoulder) and then upward (to feel the posterior shoulder); keep baby at level of uterus; vigorously stimulate infant, dry and warm; suction mouth and nose

Fast Facts

- In your triage career, you may find yourself delivering a baby in a car or waiting room. Availability of an emergency delivery tray at triage and access to bag valve masks of all sizes are imperative. Know where your supplies are and ensure they are always stocked.
- A third-trimester pregnant woman with hypotension and tachycardia or in spinal precautions needs to be positioned on her left side to aid blood return to the superior vena cava. Think in terms of meeting the needs of two patients.

Placenta Previa

1. *Questions:* Estimated due date (this condition is seen in the last trimester), vaginal bleeding (expect bright-red painless vaginal bleeding), number of pads saturating per hour?
2. *Assessment:* Palpate abdomen (expect soft abdomen and no evidence of contractions), fetal heart tones (expect within normal limits)
3. *Interventions:* Place the patient on her left side and limit exertion; anticipate the need for a pelvic ultrasound

Preeclampsia/HELLP Syndrome

1. *Questions:* Vaginal bleeding; sudden weight gain (especially if in the face); estimated due date (more than 20 weeks pregnant is high risk); right upper quadrant pain; headache, visual disturbances, or altered mental status (presence may indicate edema in brain); multiple gestation, previous hypertension, obesity, or diabetes (comorbid conditions)?
2. *Assessment:* Blood pressure greater than 140/90 mmHg (highly significant), hyperreflexia, fetal heart tones
3. *Interventions:* Anticipate the need to perform a urinalysis per protocol and expect protein in the urine; initiate seizure precaution; transfer to treatment bed and position patient on her left side

Prolapsed Cord

1. *Questions:* Sensation of the umbilical cord protruding into the vagina (often experienced after amniotic sac breaks)?
2. *Assessment:* Visualize for umbilical cord presentation
3. *Interventions:* Position immediately in knee–chest or Trendelenburg position; place sterile gloved hand in the perineal area and lift the presenting part off the cord (do not move hand until advised by physician) and anticipate emergent need for intervention

Fast Facts

Every effort should always be made to maintain the patient's dignity and privacy. An emergent presentation such as a prolapsed cord requires *immediate intervention* to potentially save the life of the baby. Lack of bed availability is not an excuse for failing to validate that in fact the cord is presenting. Acting in the best interest of the mother and baby should always come first!

Trauma in a Pregnancy Greater Than 24 Weeks

1. *Questions:* Mechanism of injury (refer to Chapter 27); vaginal bleeding or clear leaking fluid; contractions; fetal movement?
2. *Assessment:* Consider rupture of membranes and presence of leaking fluid; monitor for uterine irritability and assess fetal heart tones
3. *Interventions:* Transfer to treatment bed and position on left side; if on a backboard, tilt to the left; monitor for uterine irritability and fetal distress; anticipate the need to prepare for emergency cesarean section

Uterine Rupture

1. *Questions:* Blunt abdominal trauma; prior uterine surgery or cesarean section?
2. *Assessment:* Uterine scar; palpate for fetal parts outside the uterine cavity; hypovolemia; fetal heart tones
3. *Interventions:* Provide emotional support; anticipate labs, type and crossmatch, intravenous (IV) fluids, emergency delivery, and high likelihood of fetal demise

SPECIFIC CONDITIONS—GYNECOLOGICAL RELATED

Ovarian Torsion

1. *Questions:* Nausea and vomiting; low-grade fever; severe, sudden-onset, unilateral lower abdominal or pelvic pain; pain that

progressively worsens and radiates to groin or flank; abdominal bloating or swelling; pain with intercourse or exercise; undergoing fertility treatments; known pregnancy; previous ovarian torsion; known ovarian cyst or mass; previous pelvic surgery; history of pelvic inflammatory disease?
2. *Assessment:* Unilateral abdominal pain, unilateral rebound tenderness
3. *Intervention:* Anticipate the need for a transvaginal ultrasound and surgical intervention

Fast Facts

- A woman presenting with signs and symptoms of ovarian torsion requires rapid intervention. If the diagnosis is delayed, the ovary may become necrotic and the damage is irreversible. *Time is ovary!*
- An ectopic pregnancy is differentiated from appendicitis, as the pregnancy test is positive. Anticipate the need for an hCG blood test, as sometimes the pregnancy is too early to produce a positive urine test.

Sexual Assault

1. *Questions:* What happened, when did it happen, where do you hurt, do you know who did this to you, were there any witnesses, were weapons involved, did you or do you want to file a police report?
2. *Assessment:* Areas of injury that can be visualized at triage should be assessed and documented; perineal assessment should be deferred until a person trained in sexual assault evaluations is available; determine medical stability
3. *Interventions:* Provide emotional support and reassure the patient that she is in a safe place; line of questioning should be in private with nonjudgmental tones and gestures; notify law enforcement per jurisdiction protocols; contact the local sexual assault nurse or examiner per policy; clothing may be evidence and thus any items removed should be placed in an evidence container per protocol (e.g., paper bag), labeled as evidence with patient name, and chain of custody instituted

Fast Facts

Ask about intimate partner violence during every interaction with a pregnant woman. Since the relationship between the woman and partner changes throughout the pregnancy, this period of time places the woman at a higher risk.

Toxic Shock Syndrome

1. *Questions:* Headache or confusion; high fever that began rapidly; recent use of tampons; vomiting or diarrhea; fatigue; seizures?
2. *Assessment:* Rash (macular) with sunburn appearance that blanches with pressure; expect hypotension, tachycardia, and signs and symptoms similar to septic shock
3. *Interventions:* Initiate contact isolation precautions; position in modified Trendelenburg position; anticipate the need for rapid treatment (e.g., IV fluid, labs and blood cultures, antibiotics)

22

Behavioral Health Emergencies

Anna Sivo Montejano

Triaging a patient with a psychiatric emergency is a common occurrence in emergency facilities today. Healthcare providers need additional knowledge and resources to handle this group of patients, because they may present with unique attire and mannerisms. For example, a patient may be wearing an antenna on his head because the person believes it wards off aliens. Being compassionate and respectful and not belittling patients are important. Professional demeanor goes a long way in setting the tone for an encounter with a patient experiencing a psychiatric event. This chapter provides a foundation for potential high-acuity psychiatric presentations that the triage nurse may encounter.

Upon conclusion of this chapter, you will be able to:

1. State three worst-case scenarios of psychiatric presentation.
2. List three triage questions related to a psychiatric emergency.
3. List three "red flag" findings of psychiatric emergencies.

RED FLAG FINDINGS

- Aggressive or violent behavior
- Delusions
- Hallucinations (e.g., visual, auditory)
- Paranoia

- Patient admits to an intentional or accidental ingestion
- Patient arrives in possession of a weapon
- Patient expresses an intent or thoughts of dying or harming self or others
- Patient indicates he or she has a plan to harm self
- Speech is disorganized

WORST-CASE SCENARIOS

Danger to others, manic behavior, overdose, psychotic episode, suicide

ESSENTIAL TRIAGE QUESTIONS, ASSESSMENT, AND INTERVENTIONS

Chapter 16 is a crucial foundation for the content that follows.

Generic Questions

- What can we do for you today?
- Has anything happened recently that was different (e.g., trauma, medication noncompliance)?
- New medications?
- Any history of:
    - A traumatic loss or exposure
    - Illness or injury
    - Secondary impact (e.g., loss of job, home, financial stressors)?
- Thoughts of harming self or others?
- Is there a plan to harm self or others?
- Sleeping habits (e.g., waking up often during the night, insomnia)?

Generic Assessment

- Appearance (e.g., grooming)
- Affect, speech, behavior
- Perform a Suicide Risk Assessment; refer to https://tinyurl.com/y9pa87au for the clinical practice guideline on identifying patients at risk for suicide

Generic Interventions

- Ensure safety for patients (alone in a bathroom can be a safety issue), staff, and others.
- Remove any items that may injure the patient (e.g., belts, shoelaces, cords); place patient in a gown as soon as possible so belongings (e.g., their home medications) can be taken away and secured.
- Provide emotional support.
- Keep the patient safe by having someone watch him or her (e.g., security, sitter).

Fast Facts

- The Joint Commission National Patient Safety Goal 15 states that hospitals need to be proactive in identifying safety risks to their patient population. Any patient with a behavioral or emotional disorder requires an assessment to screen for suicide risk (The Joint Commission, 2018).
- Recognition is the first step in identifying high-risk patients so appropriate precautions can be taken.

SPECIFIC CONDITIONS

The questions, assessment, and interventions that follow are *not* intended to be comprehensive in nature but will help guide the triage nurse through the nursing process.

Danger to Others

1. *Questions:* Have you ever tried to harm someone; do you have a history of destructive behavior; do you hear voices telling you to harm others; do you have a plan to seek revenge on someone; do you have any type of weapon with you?
2. *Assessment:* Self-care; pacing, restless, unable to focus; paranoia
3. *Interventions:* Refer to Generic Interventions discussed earlier

Manic Behavior

1. *Questions:* Tell me what you are experiencing; are you sleeping?
2. *Assessment:* Unable to sit still; talkative, restless, difficulty focusing; insomnia; flight of ideas
3. *Interventions:* Orient the patient to the here and now; decrease stimuli (e.g., limit noise)

Fast Facts

- Agitated, aggressive patients are unpredictable. When escorting the patient, have the patient walk in front of you and tell him or her where to go. For example, "We are going down this hall to the room on the right." This allows you to keep your eyes on the patient and not become trapped in a corner or room where your safety is at risk.
- Patients who overdose may not be truthful. Do not worry if the "entire story" is hard to gather. Remain focused on airway, breathing, circulation, and neurological status along with vital signs and assessment.

Overdose

1. *Questions:* What did you take; how much did you take; what time did the ingestion occur (if medication was ingested, ask to see the bottle so you know the dosage and number of pills that may have been ingested); were you trying to kill yourself; why did you decide to overdose (for suspected or admitted intentional overdose); have you ever attempted to harm yourself before (if a yes response, inquire if the self-harm was an intentional overdose, etc.)?
2. *Assessment:* Refer to Generic Assessment discussed earlier in this chapter
3. *Interventions:* Obtain all medications from the patient and secure per policy; call poison control on every overdose or delegate if needed (intentional/accidental) per facility policy; think *absorption prevention* (e.g., minimize absorption of medication into the patient's body)

Psychotic Episode

1. *Questions:* Do you see or hear things that others around you do not; what do you see/hear?
2. *Assessment:* Refer to Generic Assessment discussed earlier in this chapter
3. *Interventions:* Orient patient to the here and now; provide a calm, quiet environment; reassure; do not touch patient (patients may be out of touch with reality, hallucinating, and so on, and this may frighten them)

Fast Facts

Patients may exhibit symptoms of mental illness when, in fact, the underlying issue is not behavioral health at all. The patient's final diagnosis may be thyroid storm, myxedema madness, serotonin syndrome, frontal brain tumor, neuroleptic malignant syndrome, steroid-induced psychosis, or an infection such as meningitis or encephalitis.

Suicide

1. *Questions:* Have you thought about harming yourself or others; do you have a plan to end your life; do you own a weapon; do you have anything with you right now that you can hurt yourself or others with; have you ever attempted to harm yourself; how are you sleeping?

2. *Assessment:* Self-care (e.g., hygiene)
3. *Interventions:* Refer to Generic Interventions discussed earlier

Reference

The Joint Commission. (2018). 2018 National Patient Safety Goals®. Retrieved from http://www.jointcommission.org/standards_information/npsgs.aspx

23

Ocular Emergencies

Anna Sivo Montejano and Lynn Sayre Visser

People seek medical treatment for a variety of ocular conditions. Some presentations are straightforward while others may be more complex. What is important at triage is that the nurse rapidly identifies conditions that pose a risk to loss of vision and that he or she acts with a sense of urgency. These presentations require rapid treatment and intervention in an attempt to save the eye. Time is vision! This chapter provides a foundation for potential high-acuity ocular presentations that the triage nurse may encounter.

Upon conclusion of this chapter, you will be able to:

1. State three worst-case scenarios of an ocular presentation.
2. List three triage questions related to an ocular emergency.
3. List three "red flag" findings of ocular emergencies.

RED FLAG FINDINGS

- Asymmetrical pupils(s)
- Blood in the colored part of the eye
- Chemical to the eye(s)
- Cloudy vision
- Nonreactive or diminished pupillary response
- Penetrating object to the eye(s)

- Peripheral floaters or halos around light
- Seeing red or bleeding from the eye(s) with one or more of the following: history of hypertension, bleeding disorder, trauma, or complaint of pain or change in vision
- Severe or persisting eye pain
- Steam burns to eye(s)
- Sudden onset of changes in vision
- Total, partial, or segmental loss of vision
- Toxic appearance
- Trauma to eye(s)
- Visual gaze
- Visual field as a curtain or veil

WORST-CASE SCENARIOS

Acute angle-closure glaucoma, blunt trauma to the eye(s), central retinal artery occlusion, chemical burn to the eye(s), detached retina, foreign body/corneal abrasion, orbital cellulitis, penetrating trauma to the eye(s), ruptured globe

ESSENTIAL TRIAGE QUESTIONS, ASSESSMENT, AND INTERVENTIONS

Chapter 16 is a crucial foundation for the content that follows.

Generic Questions

- Any visual disturbances (e.g., floaters, flashes of light)?
- Recent trauma (e.g., penetrating, blunt)?
- Use of eye (e.g. goggles) protection with recent activity (e.g., welding, woodworking)?
- Use of corrective lenses (e.g., glasses, contact lenses)?

Generic Assessment

- Check pupils for equal size, roundness/reactivity to light, and accommodation
- Assess eye(s) (e.g., redness, drainage, corneal changes)
- Visual acuity exam

Generic Interventions

- If sudden loss of vision is identified (e.g., partial, segmental, or total), notify the provider immediately.
- Consider the need for ocular analgesics (e.g., proparacaine) or tetanus immunization, and give nothing by mouth (NPO) if anticipating surgery.

> **Fast Facts**
>
> Patients with an ocular complaint should receive a visual acuity assessment, *but not if* they have sustained a chemical burn to the eye. For chemical burns *rapid irrigation* is the priority to halt damage to the eye.

SPECIFIC CONDITIONS

The questions, assessment, and interventions that follow are *not* intended to be comprehensive in nature but will help guide the triage nurse through the nursing process.

Acute Angle-Closure Glaucoma

1. *Questions:* Halos seen surrounding lights; cloudy vision; headache; nausea; sudden, severe unilateral eye pain; recently entered a dark room?
2. *Assessment:* Redness in eye, pupil slightly dilated and nonreactive, cornea opaque
3. *Intervention:* Notify provider immediately and anticipate the rapid need to decrease intraocular pressure

Blunt Trauma to the Eye(s)

1. *Questions:* Loss of consciousness, sudden loss of vision, trauma (consider head or neck injury)?
2. *Assessment:* Hyphema; check extraocular movements (mobility restriction due to muscle entrapment)
3. *Interventions:* Ice to injured area; place an eye shield to affected eye

Central Retinal Artery Occlusion

1. *Questions:* Sudden, painless unilateral (e.g., partial, segmental, or total) vision loss; transient vision loss; feeling of a shade coming down over the eye?
2. *Assessment:* Pupil could be dilated with a decreased response to light in affected eye
3. *Interventions:* Notify medical provider immediately, anticipate need to rapidly reestablish retinal perfusion since irreversible damage can occur within as little as 100 minutes of occlusion (Pokhrel & Loftus, 2007); have the patient breathe into a paper bag (causes vasodilation); anticipate orders for medications that lower intraocular pressure

Chemical Burns to the Eye(s)

1. *Question:* Name of agent? (Alkali agents are worse than acids and cause liquefaction necrosis.)
2. *Assessment: Do not* delay treatment to assess the patient's vision
3. *Intervention:* Anticipate the need for *immediate* irrigation of the eye; *time is vision!*

Detached Retina

1. *Questions:* Visual field has a curtain or veil; seeing floaters or flashing lights; decreased peripheral vision; history of diabetes, sickle cell, nearsightedness, or previous retinal detachment?
2. *Assessment:* Refer to Generic Assessment discussed earlier in this chapter
3. *Intervention:* Notify provider immediately since condition is time sensitive and potentially reversible

Foreign Body/Corneal Abrasion

1. *Questions:* Type of object; circumstances surrounding injury and time of injury?
2. *Assessment:* Pain may range from mild to severe
3. *Intervention:* Anticipate the need for analgesics per protocol (oral or ophthalmic)

Fast Facts

Sudden atraumatic vision loss may not always be related to the eye. The triage nurse should routinely aim to see the bigger picture and not be misled by the patient who may be convinced "it's just an eye problem." Although the patient may have an eye complaint, the more life-threatening or life-altering condition may be an evolving stroke.

Orbital Cellulitis

1. *Questions:* Recent sinus or dental infection; pain with eye movement?
2. *Assessment:* Pain with extraocular movements, impaired visual acuity (late finding); toxic appearance, fever
3. *Interventions:* Anticipate the need for a CT scan of the sinuses and orbits, laboratory tests including blood cultures, and intravenous antibiotics

Penetrating Trauma to the Eye(s)

1. *Question:* Object causing penetration (e.g., knife, pellets from a gun)?
2. *Assessment:* Refer to Generic Assessment discussed earlier in this chapter
3. *Interventions:* Place an eye shield or shields, stabilize object in place, and do not remove

Ruptured Globe

1. *Question:* History of trauma (e.g., consider blunt or penetrating trauma)?
2. *Assessment:* Pupil is teardrop in shape and deviates toward the injury; hyphema, ocular pain, blurry vision
3. *Interventions:* Do not remove any impaled objects; secure object in place; if blunt trauma occurred, patch with an eye shield; patch the unaffected eye to limit consensual eye movement; anticipate surgery

Fast Facts

- When testing visual acuity, check the affected eye first, followed by the unaffected eye, and then both eyes. If the patient is unable to read the visual acuity chart, hold fingers up and record the distance at which the patient can see your fingers; ask the patient how many fingers you are holding up. Document this information.
- If the patient cannot see the letters or fingers, check for perception of shadows or light.
- The most common complication of orbital cellulitis is meningitis.

Reference

Pokhrel, P. K., & Loftus, S. A. (2007). Ocular emergencies. *American Family Physician*, 76(6), 829–836. Retrieved from https://www.aafp.org/afp/2007/0915/p829.html

24

Musculoskeletal Emergencies

Reneé Semonin Holleran

Patients seek medical care for musculoskeletal injuries resulting from numerous causes, requiring the triage nurse to determine if the presentation extends beyond the extremity. What may initially appear as a single extremity injury may in fact meet critical trauma criteria once more in-depth questioning occurs. This chapter provides a foundation for a few high-acuity musculoskeletal presentations that the triage nurse may encounter.

Upon conclusion of this chapter, you will be able to:

1. State three worst-case scenarios of musculoskeletal presentation.
2. List three triage questions related to a musculoskeletal emergency.
3. List three "red flag" findings of musculoskeletal emergencies.

RED FLAG FINDINGS

- Extremity cyanotic and cool to touch
- High-pressure injury
- Loss of limb function and/or sensation
- Pain out of proportion to the injury
- Pulseless extremity
- Severe back pain with no history of trauma maybe indicative of a dissecting aneurysm
- Uncontrolled bleeding

WORST-CASE SCENARIOS

Amputation, arterial bleeding, arterial occlusion, compartment syndrome, high-pressure injury, neurovascular compromise (e.g., with a fracture, dislocation)

ESSENTIAL TRIAGE QUESTIONS, ASSESSMENT, AND INTERVENTIONS

Chapter 16 is a crucial foundation for the content that follows.

Generic Questions

- What happened?
- Onset (time) of symptoms/injury?
- Location of pain?
- Do you hurt anywhere else?
- Tetanus immunization history?

Generic Assessment

- Assess the six P's (pain, paresthesia, pallor, pulselessness, paralysis, poikilothermic).
- Observe for extremity deformity and check circulation, movement, and sensation.
- Inspect the site of injury and remove dressings as appropriate; palpate for crepitus.
- Note pain out of proportion to injury or history of the presenting problem.
- Assess joints above and below the area of injury or pain.
- Compare the injured extremity to the uninjured extremity.

Generic Interventions

- Initiate spinal immobilization if indicated.
- Address problems of circulation (stop the bleed—may require application of a tourniquet), airway, breathing.
- Remove jewelry or restrictive clothing from the injured extremity.
- Give nothing by mouth (NPO) if surgery/sedation is anticipated.
- Assess patient's level of pain and the need for pain management.

Fast Facts

- The patient's history of diabetes, cancer, and so on should heighten the nurse's concern and think "high risk."

SPECIFIC CONDITIONS

The questions, assessment, and interventions that follow are *not* intended to be comprehensive in nature but will help guide the triage nurse through the nursing process.

Amputation

1. *Questions:* Time of injury; location of the amputated part?
2. *Assessment:* Appearance and extent of injury; signs and symptoms of hypovolemic shock (e.g., hypotension, tachycardia)
3. *Interventions:* Apply direct pressure and place a pressure dressing to stop bleeding; anticipate the need to position patient supine if signs of shock; if the patient has brought the amputated part (e.g., finger, toe), place it in moistened sterile gauze using sterile saline (do not saturate); place the amputated part in a plastic bag or container that is securely closed, label it with the patient's information, and place the bag or container in cool water

Arterial Bleeding

1. *Questions:* Refer to Generic Questions discussed earlier in this chapter
2. *Assessment:* Estimate amount of blood loss
3. *Interventions:* Apply pressure and elevate the extremity if possible

Arterial Occlusion

1. *Questions:* History of a recent abdominal or joint replacement surgery and so on; prolonged travel (e.g., airplane, truck driver) that required sitting for an extended period of time; if a female patient, history of a recent pregnancy or delivery; pain with walking; history of prior venous thrombosis?
2. *Assessment:* Pain, pallor, cyanosis, coldness distal to occlusion, numbness, and/or paralysis
3. *Interventions:* Do not elevate or apply heat if concern for ischemic extremity; protect extremity from injury

Compartment Syndrome

1. *Questions:* Recent injury or surgical procedure to extremity?
2. Assessment: Pain out of proportion to injury
3. *Interventions:* Remove any external compression device after consulting with a physician (e.g., cast, splint); *do not* place on ice or elevate the extremity (decreases circulation); initiate NPO status; anticipate an emergent fasciotomy

> **Fast Facts**
>
> - If *pain is out of proportion* to the patient's injury or history, think compartment syndrome or, with severe back pain without history of injury, think possible ruptured aortic aneurysm.
> - When assessing circulation, always palpate a pulse distal to the injury.

High-Pressure Injury

1. *Questions:* Location of the injury; what is the substance injected (e.g., paint, grease)?
2. *Assessment:* Refer to Generic Assessment discussed earlier in this chapter
3. *Intervention:* Anticipate immediate surgical intervention (removal of the substance is vital to tissue preservation)

> **Fast Facts**
>
> - Loss of function of extremity or extremities can be indicative of a life-threatening problem.
> - Good outcomes are often dependent on timely intervention.
> - Wounds from high-pressure guns move down the sheaths of tendons and digits. Surgical intervention must be immediate so tissue can be preserved.

Neurovascular Compromise

1. *Questions:* Mechanism of injury (e.g., fall, motor vehicle crash); when did this happen; any other injuries; numbness, tingling, or decreased movement of the injured extremity; ability to ambulate?
2. *Assessment:* Palpate pulse distal to injury
3. *Interventions:* Splint in position of comfort; rest, ice, compression, and elevation (RICE); if loss of a peripheral pulse, facilitate rapid diagnostic evaluation by a medical provider; protect extremity from injury

25

Endocrine Emergencies

Dawn Friedly Gray

The endocrine system plays an important role as the messenger system of hormones and controls metabolic functioning in the body. Endocrine emergencies are usually precipitated by an acute event such as trauma, surgery, recent illness, or infection. Disruptions in normal functioning can create life-threatening emergencies and require immediate intervention. Endocrine emergencies can be difficult to detect initially because their symptoms can be vague and mimic other conditions. A good history can lead to early identification of an endocrine crisis. This chapter provides a foundation for potential life-threatening or high-risk endocrine presentations that the triage nurse may encounter.

Upon conclusion of this chapter, you will be able to:

1. State three worst-case scenarios of endocrine presentation.
2. List three triage questions related to an endocrine emergency.
3. List three "red flag" findings of endocrine emergencies.

WORST-CASE SCENARIOS

Adrenal crisis, diabetic ketoacidosis (DKA), hyperosmolar hyperglycemic state (HHS), hypoglycemia, thyroid storm

ESSENTIAL TRIAGE QUESTIONS, ASSESSMENT, AND INTERVENTIONS

Chapter 16 is a crucial foundation for the content that follows.

Generic Questions

- Onset of symptoms (gradual or abrupt)?
- Recent illness? Recent fever?
- Recent surgery?
- Past medical history?

Generic Assessment

- Vital signs
- Skin signs (skin turgor, moisture, color)
- Mental status (ranges from anxious to confused, drowsy)
- Abdominal assessment (bowel sounds, pain on palpation)

Generic Interventions

- Check glucose per protocol.
- Anticipate fluid resuscitation.
- Administer antipyretics per protocol.

SPECIFIC CONDITIONS

The questions, assessment, and interventions that follow are *not* intended to be comprehensive in nature but will help guide the triage nurse through the nursing process.

Adrenal Crisis

1. *Questions:* How long have symptoms been present; recent stressors, abrupt discontinuation of corticosteroids, recent infection, fever, nausea, vomiting, salt craving?
2. *Assessment:* Present with variety of vague symptoms; poor skin turgor, fever, appears acutely ill, vomiting; hypotension (specifically postural); generalized abdominal pain on palpation; weakness, fatigue; increased pigmentation
3. *Interventions:* Apply oxygen as needed; check glucose per protocol; anticipate electrolyte and fluid replacement and glucocorticoid administration; monitor intake and outputs (I&Os)

Fast Facts

- Presenting signs and symptoms of adrenal insufficiency can be vague and nonspecific. First diagnosis may be made when a patient presents in adrenal crisis.

Diabetic Ketoacidosis (DKA)

1. *Questions:* Recent illness, abdominal pain, nausea/vomiting; polydipsia, polyuria, polyphagia; how much insulin taken daily, when was the last dose of insulin, is there a recent blood glucose level?
2. *Assessment:* Pain on abdominal palpation (can mimic appendicitis); fruity odor to breath, Kussmaul's respirations (deep, labored, hyperventilation); poor skin turgor
3. *Interventions:* Check glucose per protocol; obtain a urinalysis to check for urine ketones; check electrolyte status especially for hypokalemia; anticipate fluid resuscitation, insulin administration, and electrolyte replacement; monitor I&Os

Hyperosmolar Hyperglycemic State (HHS)

1. *Questions:* Recent illness, polydipsia (some older adults may not have this symptom due to a decrease in their sense of thirst), polyuria?
2. *Assessment:* Poor skin turgor; tachycardia; hypotension; mental status alterations; normal respiratory status
3. *Interventions:* Check glucose per protocol; anticipate fluid resuscitation; monitor I&Os

Fast Facts

- DKA and HHS are often preceded by a precipitating event, such as infection.
- DKA has a rapid onset and blood glucose may range from 300 to 500 mg/dL. DKA presenting symptoms are often hyperventilation and abdominal pain.
- HHS has an insidious onset and serum blood glucose is 600 mg/dL or greater. HHS presents most often with neurological symptoms.

Hypoglycemia

1. *Questions:* Decreased oral intake; heavy alcohol intake; history of diabetes, insulin use, liver disease?
2. *Assessment:* Tachycardia; cool, clammy skin; tremulous; dilated pupils; confusion; seizure activity
3. *Interventions:* Check and administer glucose per protocol; administer oxygen as needed; if seizure activity, ensure seizure precautions

Fast Facts

- Since a lack of glucose may cause permanent brain dysfunction, any presentation of a patient with altered level of consciousness should have a glucose check to rule out hypoglycemia.

Thyroid Storm

1. *Questions:* Recent trauma/surgery, recent infection, thyroid medications recently discontinued, weight loss, restlessness, fever?
2. *Assessment:* Tachycardia; tachypnea; high fever; tremors; crackles secondary to heart failure; mental status changes (agitation, delirium, psychosis)
3. *Interventions:* Based on supportive care: administer oxygen as needed; cardiac monitoring; administer antipyretics and consider cooling blanket; anticipate order for beta blockers; anticipate fluid administration

26

Environmental Emergencies

Anna Sivo Montejano

The role of the triage nurse in environmental emergencies is to recognize "red flag" findings so the patient receives rapid medical treatment when indicated. The focus should be on the associated symptoms. This chapter provides a foundation for potential high-acuity environmental presentations that the triage nurse may encounter.

Upon conclusion of this chapter, you will be able to:

1. State three worst-case scenarios of an environmental presentation.
2. List three triage questions related to an environmental emergency.
3. List three "red flag" findings of environmental emergencies.

RED FLAG FINDINGS

- Altered level of consciousness
- Anaphylaxis symptoms (e.g., respiratory distress, hypotension, rash)
- Change in circulation, movement, sensation of extremities
- Chest pain, shortness of breath, dysphagia
- Core temperature: extremely low (<95°F [35°C])
- Core temperature: extremely high (>105.8°F [41°C])
- Electrical burn
- Febrile illness with systemic complaints
- Hemotoxic symptoms, such as uncontrolled bleeding

- Neurological deficits
- Neurotoxic symptoms (e.g., cognitive impairment, numb or weak extremity, visual disturbances)
- Prolonged exposure to elevated temperature combined with physical exertion or dehydration
- Seizure
- Severe muscle pain or cramping
- Severe pain
- Submersion
- Suspicion of frostbite

WORST-CASE SCENARIOS

Bites—life-threatening symptoms (e.g., animal, insect, human, snake, tick etc.), electrocution, hyperthermia, hypothermia, stings, submersion

ESSENTIAL TRIAGE QUESTIONS, ASSESSMENT, AND INTERVENTIONS

Chapter 16 is a crucial foundation for the content that follows.

Generic Questions

- Number of areas impacted (e.g., bites, stings)?
- Time of occurrence?

Generic Assessment

- Assess site of injury (e.g., puncture wounds, drainage).
- Assess circulation, movement, and sensation as indicated.
- Assess the presence of systemic complaints (e.g., abnormal vital signs).
- Determine tetanus immunization status.

Generic Interventions

- Control bleeding if observed.
- Remove jewelry or restrictive clothing from affected area.
- Apply dressings as indicated.
- Apply cold compress for animal, human, spider bite, or stings.
- Provide tetanus prophylaxis if indicated and administer per facility protocol.
- Anticipate the need for pain control and antiemetic per protocols.
- Use a marker or pen to outline borders of *localized* erythema and note date and time.

> **Fast Facts**
>
> - When assessing a wound, look for signs and symptoms of infection. Patients do not always arrive immediately after the injury occurred.
> - If it is a human or animal bite, consider taking photographs per protocol.

SPECIFIC CONDITIONS

The questions, assessment, and interventions that follow are *not* intended to be comprehensive in nature but will help guide the triage nurse through the nursing process.

Bites (Animal, Insect, Human, Tick, and Other)

1. *Questions:* What caused the bite; immunization status of animal (e.g., rabies vaccination); domesticated or nondomesticated (animal); recent hiking or camping trip?
2. *Assessment: Visualize bite site and* underlying tissue damage (e.g., nerve, blood vessel); joint involvement
3. *Interventions:* If extremity involved, immobilize and place in position of comfort; rabies vaccination as indicated per protocol (animal bite); ensure appropriate personnel follow-up with local animal control

> **Fast Facts**
>
> A cut to the knuckle sustained from punching someone in the mouth has a potential high risk of infection. Obtaining a clear history of how the injury occurred can decrease the chance of a serious infection.

Bite (Snake)

1. *Question:* Type of snake?
2. *Assessment:* Look for puncture site and monitor the patient even if no pain or swelling noted
3. *Interventions:* Minimize activity and immobilize the extremity below level of the heart to decrease blood flow to decrease uptake of venom (Hammond & Zimmermann, 2013); consider measuring the circumference of the extremity, compartment syndrome may be a complication

Electrocution

1. *Questions:* Amount of voltage (e.g., low or high); duration of contact; hearing, vision, or speech problems; concurrent trauma? Chest tightness or shortness of breath?
2. *Assessment:* Any visible burn marks, entrance or exit wounds
3. *Interventions:* Initiate basic life support measures if indicated, 12-lead ECG, dressings to visible wounds

Hyperthermia

1. *Questions:* What happened; temperature of the environment; duration of exposure; any recent physical activity, has the patient been hydrating?
2. *Assessment:* Core temperature higher than 105.8°F (41°C); nausea, vomiting, diarrhea; hot dry skin; seizures, altered level of consciousness
3. *Interventions:* Initiate basic life support measures if indicated; cooling measures immediately; rehydrate

Hypothermia

1. *Questions:* What happened; temperature of the environment; length of exposure; protective clothing worn?
2. *Assessment:* Core temperature less than 90°F (32.2°C); frostbite; burning, tingling, or numbness (fingers, toes, earlobes); waxy white color to skin or large blisters
3. *Interventions:* Initiate basic life support measures if indicated, core rewarming for a severely hypothermic patient (protect and do not rub parts that are injured); tetanus immunization per protocol

Stings

1. *Questions:* Type of sting (e.g., bee, hornet, scorpion) and the number of stings?
2. *Assessment:* Respiratory distress, chest tightness, and so on (concern for anaphylaxis); if a bee or wasp sting, assess for a visible stinger
3. *Interventions:* If able to visualize the stinger, remove using a dull object to scrape away (avoid pinching, which will release the venom)

Fast Facts

Bites to the face can result in potential airway emergencies!

Submersion

1. *Questions:* Types of water (e.g., salt, swimming pool, pond); duration of time submersed?
2. *Assessment:* Temperature (possible hypothermia); rales or wheezing
3. *Intervention:* Initiate basic life support measures if indicated

Reference

Hammond, B. B., & Zimmermann, P. G. (Eds.). (2013). *Sheehy's manual of emergency care* (7th ed.). St. Louis, MO: Mosby.

27

Trauma Emergencies

Reneé Semonin Holleran

Trauma remains one of the leading causes of death worldwide. No person is immune from the potential of trauma and, unfortunately, trauma can even cause death before birth. Despite the fact that many countries have fairly well developed emergency medical service (EMS) systems, patients who have sustained a serious injury may present for care by private vehicle. When that happens, the triage nurse needs to be ready to identify whether the patient has a life-threatening injury or injuries. This chapter provides a foundation for potential high-acuity trauma presentations that the triage nurse may encounter.

Upon conclusion of this chapter, you will be able to:

1. State three worst-case scenarios of trauma presentation.
2. List three triage questions related to a trauma emergency.
3. List three "red flag" findings of trauma emergencies.

RED FLAG FINDINGS

- Airway compromised
- Breathing difficulty/respiratory distress
- Loss of consciousness with a lucid period and is now unresponsive
- Loss of motor function
- Neurovascular compromise
- Penetrating and/or blunt injury to the head, neck, spine, chest, or abdomen

- Vital signs:
  - Glasgow Coma Scale score less than 13
  - Blood pressure less than 90 mmHg
  - Respiratory rate less than 10 or greater than 29 breaths per minute

WORST-CASE SCENARIOS

Airway, breathing, circulation, or disability impairment; blunt or penetrating trauma (head, neck, spine, chest, abdomen, extremity, pediatric, older adult); victims of violence; burns

ESSENTIAL TRIAGE QUESTIONS, ASSESSMENT, AND INTERVENTIONS

Chapter 16 is a crucial foundation for the content that follows. In addition, an awareness of trauma criteria, which include physiological, anatomical, and mechanism of injury, is imperative for the triage nurse to determine the appropriate level of care for the patient. Not all criteria can be discussed in this chapter but mechanism of injury is elaborated upon because this is more commonly seen in triage. The importance of posting trauma criteria in the triage area cannot be overemphasized. The ability to reference information quickly can make a difference in assigning the appropriate acuity level. Information about trauma criteria can be located at www.cdc.gov/mmwr/pdf/rr/rr6101.pdf.

Generic Questions

- Use trauma criteria (physiological [especially blood pressure, pulse, and respirations], anatomical, and mechanism of injury) to facilitate line of questioning.

Mechanism of Injury

- Motor vehicle crash: Events surrounding the vehicle crash (restrained vs. unrestrained, ejected, high speed [>60 mph (97 kph)], death in same vehicle, rollover, prolonged extrication [>30 minutes], and age of the patient [pediatric, adult, older adult])?
- Involved in an explosion?
- Motor vehicle/cyclist impact greater than 30 mph (48 kph)?
- Pedestrian impact?
- Fall: Adult fall greater than 15 ft (4.6 m); pediatric fall greater than 10 ft (3 m)?
- Penetrating injury (e.g., gunshot, stabbing): Location on the body?

Generic Assessment

Airway

- Inability to protect his or her airway; presence of blood or vomitus in the airway; if airway manipulated, remember cervical spine immobilization

Breathing

- Absent, slow, or labored (e.g., accessory muscle use, retractions, nasal flaring)

Circulation

- Pulseless, bradycardic or tachycardic, decreased or absent peripheral pulses (check all extremities), pale and diaphoretic, pulse less than 50 bpm or greater than 100 bpm (pediatrics greater than 120 bpm), uncontrolled bleeding

Disability

- Unconscious, altered mental status, loss of function of any extremity or extremities, clear fluid mixed with blood from nose or ears, nausea and vomiting, suspected spinal cord injury

Injuries

- *Blunt Injuries:* Significant injury to a single region (e.g., head, neck, chest, abdomen, axilla, groin) or injury to two or more regions of the body; visible signs of blunt trauma
- *Penetrating Injuries:* Head, neck, spine, chest, abdomen, pelvis, groin, and axilla
- *Orthopedic Injuries:* Limb amputations and limb-threatening injuries, including loss of a peripheral pulse or a cold or cyanotic limb; serious crush injury; major compound fracture or open dislocation; fractured pelvis; fractures of two or more of the following: femur, tibia, and humerus; signs of shock related to these injuries

History

- Obtain a **SAMPLE** History

    Symptoms

    Allergies

    Medications

    Past medical history

    Last oral intake

    Events preceding the incident

Generic Interventions

- Act on any airway, breathing, circulation, disability, or environmental/exposure impairment.
  - *Airway:* Open the airway with cervical spine protection and suction any blood or vomitus if present; initiate basic life support protocols if indicated.
  - *Breathing:* Assist with ventilations as needed with bag valve mask. Place patient on high-flow oxygen; allow patient to assume a position of comfort while protecting the cervical spine.
  - *Circulation:* Initiate basic life support protocols if indicated; manage any uncontrolled bleeding, making sure of the availability of a method to manage bleeding, including a tourniquet or a commercial stop-the-bleeding kit.
  - *Disability:* Assess level of consciousness.
  - *Environmental/Exposure:* Remove any clothing that may be contaminated (e.g., fuel) or interfering with breathing or circulation, and keep the patient warm.
- Decide which level of care the patient may require, for example, a trauma surgeon or care in the general ED.

Fast Facts

- If the triage nurse identifies a patient with a potential cervical spine injury who arrives by private vehicle, ambulates into triage, or is carried in the arms of another person, knowing where the supplies (e.g., cervical collar, backboard) are kept for immediate access is necessary. Calling for assistance from the local EMS agency may be essential if extrication poses a challenge.
- Safety of the staff, patient, and others should always be the primary concern when managing a patient who has sustained an injury, especially one that is the result of violence.

CONDITION-SPECIFIC QUESTIONS RELATED TO TRAUMA

For the following worst-case scenarios, refer to the generic questions, assessment, and interventions discussed earlier in this chapter for further information.

Abdominal Trauma

- *Questions:* Mechanism of injury (e.g., blunt or penetrating); abdominal pain and, if so, where; any referred pain (e.g., shoulder pain, which could indicate a liver or splenic injury); nausea or vomiting; difficulty urinating or hematuria; obvious signs of injury (e.g., open wounds or seat belt sign); patient more than 20 weeks pregnant?

Chest Trauma

- *Questions:* Mechanism of injury (e.g., blunt or penetrating); respiratory distress; obvious signs of injury (e.g., open wounds, seat belt sign)?

Extremity Trauma

- *Questions:* Open fracture or any open wounds near the injury, loss of function in the extremity, numbness or tingling in the extremity, loss of peripheral pulse?

Head Trauma

- *Questions:* History of loss of consciousness, and if so, how long; was there a period of "lucidity" and then a change in mental status; has patient taken anything (alcohol or drugs) that may have altered his or her mental status?

Spinal Trauma

- *Questions:* Able to move all his or her extremities; any weakness; any complaints of neck pain, numbness, or weakness?

Older Adult Trauma

- *Questions:* What medications is the patient taking; what other medical problems does the patient have (e.g., diabetes, chronic obstructive pulmonary disease [COPD]); known history of cognitive impairment?

Pediatric Trauma

- *Questions:* Was an appropriate restraint device used (if in a vehicle), abnormal behaviors, parent concerned about any changes in the child?

Fast Facts

Knowing which patients may be at a higher risk after sustaining a traumatic injury increases the nurse's awareness of a potentially worsening scenario:
- Age risk (younger than 5 or older than 55 years)
- Comorbidities: diabetes, COPD, cardiac disease, and so on

(continued)

(*continued*)

- Poor general impression of the patient: "Looks like something is wrong"
- Victims of violence: sexual assault, domestic violence, child maltreatment
- Pregnancy of greater than 20 weeks gestation
- Severe pain

Victims of Violence

- *Questions:* Does the injury match the history or mechanism of injury, are you and the patient safe, is the patient intoxicated, is the patient accompanied by law enforcement, was the patient restrained during the violent act?

Fast Facts

- When taking care of victims of violence, speak in a calm voice and ensure that it is safe for you and the team to approach the patient.
- Clothing and personal belongings may be used as evidence.
- Handle each piece of evidence with a new pair of gloves to prevent cross-contamination.
- Cut clothing in such a way to preserve evidence.
- Place items in an evidence container per protocol (e.g., paper bag).
- Use extreme caution when searching a patient who has been involved in a violent incident.
- Give weapons or evidence (labeled with the patient's name, date of collection) to the appropriate authorities or store in a safe secured area.

Burns

- *Question:* Has the patient inhaled any smoke or chemicals or been in a fire in an enclosed-space?
- *Assessment:* Signs of inhalation injury, including facial burns, singed nasal or facial hair, hoarse voice; burns over a large area of the patient's body (greater than 20%) or burns to the hands or feet
- *Interventions:* Ensure that it is safe to approach the patient; patients with chemical burns may need to be taken directly to a decontamination area; use appropriate personal protective equipment; manage the patient's airway, breathing, circulation, and disability; remove all clothing and jewelry to stop the burning process

28

Infectious Presentations

Anna Sivo Montejano and Lynn Sayre Visser

Patients with contagious illnesses who seek care may manifest a variety of signs and symptoms, often including dermal findings, which can be challenging to evaluate. The triage nurse's role is not to diagnose the rash but rather to ensure that the patient's airway, breathing, and circulation (ABC) are intact and that patients with potentially contagious conditions are identified and appropriately isolated. This chapter focuses on many conditions that are a high priority for isolation in order to protect the patient, staff, and those waiting.

Upon conclusion of this chapter, you will be able to:

1. State three contagious conditions.
2. List three triage questions related to a dermal presentation.
3. List three "red flag" findings of dermal presentations.

RED FLAG FINDINGS

- Evidence of dehydration if immunocompromised
- Facial or tongue edema
- Mental status changes (confusion or decreased level of consciousness)
- New-onset petechiae or purpura with or without a fever
- Rapid progression of symptoms or rash
- Rash near the eye or vision changes
- Rash with severe headache, stiff neck, or fever

- Recent break in the skin with rapid-onset progression (e.g., necrotizing fasciitis)
- Severe pain or itching
- Swelling and redness located near or around eye(s), over joints, or in the genital region
- Symptomatic with prior history of severe allergic reaction
- Systemic complaints: near syncope, dizziness, shortness of breath, weakness, or nausea and vomiting
- Throat swelling, stridor, or drooling (new onset)
- Wheezing, shortness of breath, or chest pain

INFECTIOUS PRESENTATIONS

Chickenpox, impetigo, lice, measles, meningitis, rubella, scabies, shingles, smallpox (a bioterrorist hazard)

ESSENTIAL TRIAGE QUESTIONS, ASSESSMENT, AND INTERVENTIONS

Chapter 16 is a crucial foundation for the content that follows.

Generic Questions

- Location of rash, wound, or inflamed area? (Ask about genitalia; the patient may not tell you.)
- Pattern of rash presentation (e.g., begins on head first vs. hands or feet)?
- Fever or sore throat?
- New detergent, medication, food, or chemical exposure?
- Exposure to others with a similar rash or anyone living in the same household with the rash?
- Previous rash or hives (and the cause)?
- School outbreak of a rash (e.g., scabies, lice)?
- Recent exposure to a person with a communicable disease?
- Recent travel (e.g., another country or region)?
- Immunization status: diphtheria, tetanus, and pertussis (DTaP); varicella (chickenpox); measles, mumps, and rubella (MMR); influenza; pneumococcal vaccine (PCV)?

Fast Facts

- On September 30, 2014, the first case of Ebola virus disease was diagnosed in the United States in a man who had recently arrived from Liberia. In the following weeks, two healthcare workers who cared for the patient contracted the disease and many other

(continued)

(continued)

individuals were regularly monitored for symptoms. In 2018 an outbreak in the Democratic Republic of Congo occurred, again bringing attention to this potentially deadly disease. These cases are a reminder to all healthcare workers that we must *always* be vigilant in assessing a patient's *travel history* in addition to questioning about symptoms, including fever of unknown origin. Centers for Disease Control and Prevention (CDC) guidelines and facility protocols should always be followed.

Generic Assessment

- Characteristics of rash
  - Extent of rash
  - Appearance (e.g., macular, papular, vesicular, hives)
  - Color (e.g., red, blanchable/nonblanchable)
  - Distribution pattern (e.g., symmetrical/asymmetrical)
  - Examine hands and feet (may provide information that helps identify the rash)
- Check mucous membranes for dehydration (e.g., mouth, eyes)

Generic Interventions

- Wear gloves while assessing patient to avoid contact with his or her skin or clothing
- Apply dressings for draining wounds
- Consider initiation of appropriate isolation for patient, staff, and visitors (e.g., airborne, droplet, contact) and use appropriate personal protective equipment
- Isolate patient if suspicion of an infectious presentation
  - Airborne precautions (e.g., negative pressure room, room with a high-efficiency particulate air filter); mask patient until placed in negative pressure room
    - Chickenpox/shingles (both airborne and contact precautions)
    - Smallpox (both airborne and contact precautions)
  - Droplet precautions: mumps, rubella (German measles), measles (rubeola)
  - Contact precautions: lice, scabies, impetigo, smallpox, chickenpox/shingles

Fast Facts

- Focus on the symptoms and nursing interventions *first*. If the dermatological findings seem allergy related, identifying the allergen is secondary to treating the patient.

(continued)

(continued)

- Rapid progression of a rash places a patient at higher risk for a severe respiratory condition and possible anaphylaxis.
- Early recognition of Stevens–Johnson syndrome and toxic epidermal necrolysis can result in quick, appropriate care. The patient may complain of a burning rash that begins on the face and upper torso, and skin can be noted to peel off in sheets. This patient presentation requires reverse isolation to prevent infection.

CONDITIONS REQUIRING ISOLATION

Many presentations require isolation to prevent exposure of other patients, visitors, and staff. The following discussion is *not* all encompassing but provides information that may help the triage nurse understand rash progression, determine when to initiate isolation, and guide triage decision-making. For additional information, see www.cdc.gov.

- *Chickenpox:* Occurs in individuals with a recent exposure to someone with chickenpox; patient may or may not present with a rash since patient is contagious 48 hours before rash erupts and remains contagious until lesions crust over; incubation period is 10 to 21 days after exposure to chickenpox (CDC, 2016); rash appears first on the face, back, or abdomen and then spreads; rash starts as small red bumps (pimples) that develop into blisters and has varying stages of eruption; may have signs of dehydration from sores in mouth (due to difficulty swallowing fluids)
- *Impetigo:* Exposure to a person with impetigo; contagious until lesions crust over; rash to the lips, face, legs, or arms and spreads easily; itchy blisters filled with yellowish fluid
- *Lice:* Rash mostly found on the scalp and behind ears, and patient feels movement on scalp (head lice); rash presents on waist, thighs, and groin (body lice)
- *Measles (Rubeola):* Recent exposure to a person with measles; incubation period is 10 to 12 days with rash appearing approximately 14 days after exposure; patient is contagious 4 days before rash erupts and it continues for 4 days after the rash appears (CDC, 2017); rash starts on the head before spreading to most of the body, including hands and feet; three Cs include cough, conjunctivitis, coryza (runny nose); Koplik (white) spots inside the mouth; causes itching; rash is said to "stain" the skin, changing from red to dark brown before disappearing (easier to see in light-skinned people)

- *Meningitis:* There are many types of meningitis; the bacterial type can be life threatening, which is spread from person to person in a variety of ways, such as sharing food, coughing, or kissing; risks are large groups of people (college campuses), traveling out of the country to certain locations, and certain medical conditions; signs and symptoms are nausea, vomiting, confusion, photophobia, and so on; if you suspect meningitis, notify a medical provider immediately, in only a few hours, death can occur (CDC, 2018a)
- *Rubella:* Recent exposure to a person with rubella; incubation period for 14 days after exposure; rash is first identified on the face and spreads to the chest, back, and limbs; lesions are in different stages of development; begins with fever, runny nose, and cough followed by characteristic rash; itchy
- *Scabies:* Rash often found in the webs of fingers, wrists, belt or bra line, and buttocks; small black dot at the center of rash; severe itching; symptoms may not develop for 4 to 6 weeks after an exposure to scabies; patient can be contagious even before symptoms develop (CDC, 2018b)
- *Shingles:* Occurs in individuals with a history of chickenpox; patient is contagious until the lesions crust over, rash does not cross the midline (follows a dermatome), extremely painful

Fast Facts

Shingles often only appear in one patch (along one dermatome), but if the rash is present along three or more dermatomes the nurse should be highly suspicious that the patient is immunocompromised (e.g., cancer, HIV infection, recent transplant, taking immune suppressant medications). Shingles can include involvement of the central nervous system and may lead to potentially fatal encephalitis (CDC, 2018c).

- *Smallpox:* Incubation period is 12 to 14 days; first week of the rash is the most contagious period; rash erupts first in the mouth, followed by a rash to the arms and legs, and later hands, feet, and other parts of the body; rash erupts all at once and appears uniform in size and shape; accompanied by fever, vomiting, malaise, and head and body aches

Fast Facts

- Does the patient have pain that lessens 24 to 36 hours after an injury and then rapidly worsens? Think necrotizing fasciitis, commonly known as *flesh-eating disease*. Symptoms

(continued)

(continued)

tend to be rapidly progressive and may include fever, chills, nausea, and malaise. Approximately 25% of people with this condition will die (National Necrotizing Fasciitis Foundation, 2018).
- Patients at risk for necrotizing fasciitis include those with a recent break in the skin (e.g., from surgical procedure, wound, or intravenous drug use), diabetes, immunosuppression, or a history of malignancy.
- The patient assessment may reveal *pain out of proportion* to what is visible on the skin and crepitus due to the release of toxins as tissue is being destroyed. Upon initial presentation, the wound may or may not appear infected, but after 3 to 4 days the area of injury may appear purplish or necrotic (National Necrotizing Fasciitis Foundation, 2018).
- Although necrotizing fasciitis is *not* a contagious condition, a presentation of a reddened or purplish area with an accompanying fever should always cause the triage nurse to *consider* the need for isolation.
- Nursing interventions include anticipating the need for rapid medical or surgical intervention, antibiotics, and use of a marker or pen to outline borders of localized erythema and mark with date and time. Marking the skin helps staff closely monitor the progression of the area of concern.

References

Centers for Disease Control and Prevention. (2016). Chickenpox (varicella). Retrieved from https://www.cdc.gov/chickenpox

Centers for Disease Control and Prevention. (2017). Transmission of measles. Retrieved from https://www.cdc.gov/measles/about/transmission.html

Centers for Disease Control and Prevention. (2018a). Meningitis. Retrieved from https://www.cdc.gov/meningitis/index.html

Centers for Disease Control and Prevention. (2018b). Scabies frequently asked questions (FAQs). Retrieved from https://www.cdc.gov/parasites/scabies/gen_info/faqs.html

Centers for Disease Control and Prevention. (2018c). Shingles (herpes zoster). Retrieved from https://www.cdc.gov/shingles

National Necrotizing Fasciitis Foundation. (2018). The symptoms of NF. Retrieved from http://www.nnff.com/the-symptoms-of-nf.html

VI

Special Considerations in Triage Nursing

29

Special Populations in Triage

Anna Sivo Montejano

Patients come to healthcare facilities seeking medical treatment. As triage nurses, our job is to assess them thoroughly, determine treatment needs, and direct them to the most appropriate treatment area. What happens when the patient has special considerations such as a hearing, visual, or cognitive impairment? Perhaps there is a language barrier, or the patient is a member of the military who requires special attention. How easy is it to thoroughly assess them and make sure that nothing is overlooked? Awareness of these considerations can make the difference in whether the patient receives the most appropriate care. This chapter focuses on groups of individuals who may get overlooked.

Upon conclusion of this chapter, you will be able to:

1. State three special populations seen by triage nurses.
2. List three suggestions for recognizing a victim of sex trafficking (ST).
3. List two suggestions to improve communication with developmentally delayed patients.

HUMAN TRAFFICKING

Although human trafficking is not an activity one would expect to encounter in the United States, sadly this problem is becoming more common. The term *human trafficking* can refer to sex trafficking, commercial sexual exploitation (CSE), or child sex trafficking (CST).

The vulnerability of children puts them at particular risk for this type of abuse. Victims are exposed to oppressive exploitation and physical and mental harm. Providing their "service" up to 12 hours a day results in physical injuries, sexually transmitted diseases (STDs), malnutrition, isolation, and psychological trauma. What can a triage nurse do to stop this horrific abuse? *Recognize* that this exists, *intervene* appropriately, and *refer* (Miller, 2013).

Suggestions for Recognizing the Victim

- Individual is accompanied by a person who stays close and speaks for him or her
- Individual lies about his or her age
- May have multiple differing forms of identification
- Inconsistencies or denial of injuries and illnesses, patient/keeper often changing stories
- Individual does not have possession of his or her own documents (e.g., passport, birth certificate)
- Presence of STDs, yeast or bacterial infections, particularly in underage patients
- Highly anxious or obedient demeanor (Miller, 2013)
- Trafficker is often the same nationality as the victim
- Presence of tattoo that may be a number, a symbol, or the trafficker's initials (shows ownership)
- Bald patches (e.g., hair being pulled out)
- Presence of a global positioning system (GPS) tracking bracelet (Peters, 2013)

One must be sensitive to what the victim is enduring on a day-to-day basis in a world with no hope of escape. Victims are often told by their traffickers that no one is there for them and they are alone. Consequently, they may have a distrust of others that incapacitates them.

Victims may exhibit:

- Fear and distrust related to possible imprisonment or deportation
- Shame
- Lack of emotion or, conversely, intense anger
- A strong attachment to the trafficker
- Anger toward the nurse or other healthcare professionals (e.g., the victim may fear that questions will upset the trafficker)
- Limited communication ability as they may not speak English
- Feelings of depression or possible suicidal ideation (Peters, 2013)

Tips for the Nurse

- Recognize behaviors that are characteristic of victims.
- Talk to the victim *alone*.

- Keep the victim and staff safe; interfering with the trafficker's "property" can result in an unsafe situation.
- Notify security, local police, or both.

A triage nurse's *awareness* is our first line of defense. With this knowledge and the passion to help the victims of this unimaginable slavery, we can make a difference in the lives of those who may not have come to the attention of victim advocates or child protective services in our communities. Do not think this issue exists only in faraway places. These individuals can be living in your community at this very moment.

Fast Facts

- Be mindful that a relative of the victim may be the trafficker. Trust your instincts!
- The triage nurse must *look beneath the surface*. Every minute, every day, every patient could be a victim of sex trafficking (Peters, 2013).

INTIMATE PARTNER VIOLENCE

Intimate partner violence (IPV), sometimes referred to as domestic violence, is an act in which the victim is assaulted by his or her intimate partner. The assaultive act may come in many forms, and you may encounter a combination of these forms together.

- Physical
- Emotional
- Financial
- Sexual
- Psychological

Recognition seems like it would be easy when one out of every three women have experienced physical violence from their intimate partners in their lifetime (Black et al., 2011). The National Coalition Against Domestic Violence (n.d.) reports that in the United States, on an average close to 20 persons per minute are physically abused by their intimate partner. Abuse affects not only women but also teenagers, men, partners in same-sex relationships, and bisexual and transgender couples. Recognition is the first step in helping victims of IPV.

Every patient needs to be screened appropriately because IPV is found in all of the following groups:

- Ethnicity
- Religious

- Economic
- Age
- Educational

The triage nurse must ask questions regarding the potential victim's safety, but the key is making these inquiries privately. If questions are asked in a safe environment and in a nonjudgmental fashion, the victim is more likely to be forthcoming about the history of the violence.

Sometimes the aggressor partner will not leave the victim's side, making it challenging to screen the victim. Explain to the patient that a urine specimen is needed, or an x-ray, thus separating the potential victim from the partner, in a location where the partner may not follow. This is your opportunity to ask the victim if he or she feels safe. Once IPV is identified, take action and adhere to your facility policies. Remember: you can make a difference in saving the life of a victim, but you must first ask the question.

MILITARY PERSONNEL

Being culturally competent in nursing has been a necessary ingredient to better understand the needs and values of patients of different ethnicities, socioeconomic status, religions, and so on, but we must not overlook another special population—our military personnel. The military culture focuses on loyalty, selflessness, and following moral codes. Nurses must be aware of the risk factors that military men and women are prone to so interventions can be timely and accurate.

Most Common Chief Complaints

- Musculoskeletal conditions (most common are back, ankle/knee, and shoulder pain)
- Postsurgical complications
- Behavioral health issues (e.g., depression, post-traumatic stress disorder, suicide)

The heightened awareness can assist nurses in asking appropriate questions and being aware of signs that might otherwise go unnoticed. The nurse may wonder, "Why does not the patient just tell me the real reason for the visit?" From a military perspective, a potential behavioral health problem may serve as a major barrier to obtaining care.

When it comes to amputations, direct communication about their loss of limb is appropriate. They are aware the limb is gone. These individuals have already undergone surgery, physical and occupational rehabilitation, as well as psychological therapy. Providers who have little experience in providing care to these individuals find direct communication difficult. It is common for the veteran to comment or make jokes about the limb. For example, one veteran, having lost three limbs and undergone multiple abdominal surgeries, wore a T-shirt to the ED saying "combat veteran, some assembly required."

Indications of Military Personnel (Former or Current)

- Tattoo of an anchor, eagle, or globe
- Tattoo around the wrist (like a bracelet), on the deltoid(s) forearm, or chest signifies a fallen comrade(s)
- Addressing others as "sir" or "ma'am"
- Clothing
- Body language
- Making direct eye contact

When triaging a military member, active or retired, who presents with a behavioral health complaint, the healthcare provider needs to maintain situational awareness. Active or veteran military members commonly carry sidearms (weapons) in public. Part of the triage assessment is to ask the patient and/or family if the individual is carrying a weapon. Do not attempt to take the weapon from the individual but rather contact security or your local police department for assistance.

Fast Facts

Do not hesitate to ask patients if they have been or are associated with the military. Such a simple question may make a difference in getting a patient the care he or she truly needs.

LESBIAN, GAY, BISEXUAL, TRANSGENDER, QUESTIONING/QUEER (LGBTQ) PATIENTS

The transgender population often delays seeking treatment because of their past experience with healthcare providers, often described as unprofessional, biased, negative, harassing, and unwelcoming. Sadly the patient's delay in treatment can lead to a worsening of his or her illness (Grossman, 2016).

Suggestions when assessing a LGBTQ patient include:

- Stay focused on the reason for the patient's visit.
- Be nonjudgmental.
- Listen to how the patient self-identifies with himself/herself (pay attention to the pronoun being used).

- If something is said incorrectly, do not overapologize.
- If you are unsure regarding how to address your patient, be respectful and just ask what the patient prefers.

As healthcare providers, we must be caring and compassionate to all patients we encounter in our line of work. Being respectful and compassionate goes a long way in the care of patients.

LEFT VENTRICULAR ASSIST DEVICE PATIENTS

Healthcare providers are encountering left ventricular assist devices (LVADs) more often among patients with heart failure who are awaiting a heart transplant or other cardiac conditions. Years ago these patients needed to remain hospitalized, but now these devices use battery packs that allow the patients to remain mobile. As triage nurses, we need to be familiar with the potential complications of these devices.

Complications in LVAD Patients

- Infection
- Thromboemboli
- Device malfunction
- Right-sided heart failure
- Hemolysis

Although knowing the potential complications is important, having a basic knowledge of the normal findings for an LVAD patient is also vital when completing an assessment.

Normal Findings in LVAD Patients

- Pulses are usually absent
- Systolic blood pressure (SBP) range of 70 to 90 mmHg via Doppler reading
- Ventricular assist devices (VADs) may "hum" loudly
- Be aware that these patients are on anticoagulation therapy

The nurse must be familiar with the LVAD and understand the resources available to troubleshoot the device, such as who and what phone number to call if in need of help with the device.

Suggestions to Assist LVAD Patients

- When assessing the patient, if there is concern about the device malfunctioning, contact the LVAD center listed on the patient's VAD card (carried by the patient at all times).
- If you hear beeps or alarms, refer to the symbols displayed and call the number on the patient's VAD card.

- If you need to assist with defibrillation or cardioversion, place the external patches, one anteriorly and one posteriorly.
- Cardiopulmonary resuscitation (CPR) should be performed only upon confirming LVAD malfunction.

HEARING-IMPAIRED PATIENTS

When patients with a hearing impairment arrive at a healthcare facility, we need to do our best to complete an accurate assessment. Simultaneously, we need to provide an environment in which patients feel their impairment is not affecting their ability to express their concerns and one in which our ability to understand them is not hindered.

Suggestions to Assist the Hearing Impaired

- Offer a certified sign language interpreter.
- If the patient has arrived with a person to "interpret or be their eyes," allow this person to accompany them as much as possible.
- Use a paper and pen.
- Have patients lip-read if they state that is acceptable to them.
- Pay close attention to nonverbal communication.
- If hearing aid(s) are being worn, ensure proper placement and function.
- Use a text-telephone device (TTD) or telecommunication device for the deaf (TDD).

VISUALLY IMPAIRED PATIENTS

A patient who is visually impaired requires the triage nurse to adapt the triage processes. Nurses may think they need to talk loudly so the patient can hear them. The patient is not deaf, so speaking in a normal tone when communicating is appreciated. Making patients feel comfortable when they cannot see their surroundings is an important part of reducing patients' anxiety in an unfamiliar environment.

Suggestions to Assist the Visually Impaired

- Introduce yourself and let the patient know everything you are doing; for example, "I am going to get a urine specimen cup for you."
- Ask patients if they need help before assuming they do.
- Ask if the patient uses any visual aid, such as a cane or service animal (if not present with them).
- Guide patients to where you need them to go by letting them hold onto your arm.

- Let patients know how they can find you for any questions or concerns (e.g., if they are sitting in the waiting room, walk them to the front desk so they know where to find assistance).
- Update the patient verbally because the visual clues are not available.
- Introduce every new individual involved in the patient's care; remember that he or she cannot see who enters the room.
- If you leave the room, verbally tell the patient.
- Ask patients where they would like their belongings so they know where to find them if an item is needed.
- Make sure all their questions are answered and needs are met.

ILLITERATE PATIENTS

An illiterate patient does not have the ability to read or write, which may not be evident initially at triage. However, paying close attention to nonverbal signs may provide clues. As triage nurses, we must clarify with patients, in a nondemeaning way, whether they can read and write. Not following through when there is a suspicion of illiteracy can have detrimental implications because the patient cannot understand written instructions.

Suggestions to Assist the Illiterate Population

- Have the patient give you a return demonstration or verbalize key elements of discharge instructions.
- Draw pictures to help with explanations or instructions.
- Use pictures and pain scales (e.g., Wong–Baker) with assessments.

LANGUAGE BARRIER PATIENTS

Many languages are spoken in the United States today. With patients and visitors originating from all areas of the world, ensuring effective communication is vital. Treating each person as a unique individual and being respectful of differing beliefs can aid in recovery.

Suggestions to Assist Patients With a Language Barrier

- Ensure that a certified interpreter is provided.
  - Some facilities have in-house translation services.
- Use a phone with two handsets so the patient and healthcare provider can be on the phone at the same time as the interpreter.
- Utilize picture boards.

Although convenient, avoid having family members act as interpreters. They may not accurately relay questions to the patient or convey all the information you provide, information may be of a personal nature, or maltreatment may be a possibility.

DEVELOPMENTALLY DELAYED, AUTISTIC, OR THE LIKE PATIENTS

When a patient who is developmentally delayed or autistic arrives at your facility, how do you ascertain his or her level of knowledge? Where do you begin? How do you elicit the true story of the patient's visit? Healthcare providers are sometimes uncomfortable interviewing patients who are developmentally delayed, autistic, or the like. They may worry that important information may be missed, resulting in a detrimental outcome. In such situations, nurses must be careful not to make assumptions. Family members, caretakers, and others who know the patient can help the nurse understand the patient's baseline function, assisting the nurse in performing an accurate triage assessment. The individuals who spend time with these patients know them best.

Suggestions to Assist the Developmentally Delayed, Autistic, or the Like

- Ask the accompanying person about the patient's baseline function.
- Inquire about any changes the caretaker is concerned about.
- Ask simple questions and move slowly.
- Explain to the patient what you are doing.
- Pay very close attention to nonverbal signs.
- Always be cognizant of the possibility of maltreatment.

Fast Facts

Patience is essential when meeting the needs of unique groups of people. Patients may not always understand what is going on in their immediate surroundings. Your patience and kindness can go a long way in facilitating the patient–provider encounter.

References

Black, M. C., Basile, K. C., Breiding, M. J., Smith, S. G., Walters, M. L., Merrick, M. T., . . . Stevens, M. R. (2011). *The National Intimate Partner and Sexual Violence Survey (NISVS): 2010 summary report*. Atlanta, GA: National Center for Injury Prevention and Control, Centers for Disease Control and Prevention. Retrieved from http://www.cdc.gov/violenceprevention/pdf/nisvs_executive_summary-a.pdf

Grossman, V. G. (2016). Providing quality care to the transgender patient in the radiology setting. *Journal of Radiology Nursing, 35*(3), 218–226. doi:10.1016/j.jradnu.2016.06.002

Miller, C. L. (2013). Child sex trafficking in the emergency department: Opportunities and challenges. *Journal of Emergency Nursing, 39*(5), 477–478. doi:10.1016/j.jen.2013.06.004

National Coalition Against Domestic Violence. (n.d.). Statistics. Retrieved from https://ncadv.org/statistics

Peters, K. (2013). The growing business of human trafficking and the power of emergency nurses to stop it. *Journal of Emergency Nursing, 39*(3), 280–288. doi:10.1016/j.jen.2012.03.017

30

Pediatric Triage

Deb Jeffries

Wherever you may be working, being prepared to care for a pediatric patient is crucial. Triage of pediatric patients can be intimidating for even the experienced nurse. Accurately triaging pediatric patients will require every bit of knowledge and expertise you possess with a little ingenuity thrown in. Always remember when caring for children, you really have two patients: the child and the caregiver. This chapter covers an overview of pediatric patients and their developmental stages along with some triage perils.

Upon conclusion of this chapter, you will be able to:

1. State two high-risk pediatric presentations.
2. Verbalize effective methods of communication with pediatric patients of varying developmental stages.
3. Explain special considerations when triaging pediatric patients.

PEDIATRIC TRIAGE: OVERVIEW

In spite of the challenges associated with triage of the pediatric patient, you are much more likely to make sound decisions if you fully embrace a critical concept: *Listen!*

- That's right: *Listen* to the parents or caregivers and fight with every ounce within you the temptation to categorize them as *overreacting*. Although you have no doubt heard it said that "parents know their

child much better than you do," it bears repeating here: "Parents know their child much better than you do!"
- *Listen* to the child. If children are verbal, give weight to their words and learn developmental stages so that you will be able to communicate effectively with those of various ages. If they are nonverbal, *listen* and pay careful attention to the intensity and pitch of their cry *and identify whether or not they are consolable.*
- *Listen* to your colleagues. Use the resources available to you whenever you are not comfortable with a presentation or are not sure what to do.
- *Listen* to the medical providers; ask questions. Often providers not only want to collaborate with nurses, they want to teach us, allowing us to become more expert.
- *Listen* to yourself. If your intuition "tells" you the child in front of you is sicker than the medical record appears to indicate, then do something about it and get that child in front of a provider.

DEVELOPMENTAL STAGES

Familiarity with developmental stages is a *must*! You cannot recognize abnormal findings if you do not know what normal is! While a full discussion of this topic is beyond the scope of this book, information applicable to triage assessments of children in different developmental stages follows:

Infant (Birth–1 year)
- *Trust versus mistrust:* Separation fears begin at about 6 months; period of greatest growth; improving motor skills, from lifting head to standing

Toddler (1–3 years)
- *Autonomy versus shame and doubt:* Likes the word *no*; separation fears continue; risk takers; negotiation with a toddler is not effective (*tip:* be friendly but firm!); allow child to remain with caregiver whenever possible; anterior fontanelles close at 18 to 24 months

Preschooler (3–5 years)
- *Initiative versus shame and guilt:* Magical thinking is common; illness is sometimes seen as punishment; allow child the opportunity to ask questions; may want to dress/undress self

School Age (6–12 years)
- *Industry versus inferiority:* Takes pride in accomplishments (*tip:* offer praise frequently); able to think logically (*tip:* explain what you are doing!)

Adolescent (13–18 years)
- *Identity versus role confusion:* Independent, moody, risk takers (*tip:* allow them to have options whenever possible); excessively modest, despite their appearance (*tip:* provide privacy when the patient is getting undressed; Newman & Newman, 2014)

Fast Facts

- Communicating a caring attitude toward a child will make obtaining information from the parent or caregiver much easier. If a parent senses the nurse's frustration or lack of patience during the interaction, the subjective assessment will be much harder!
- It has been said that a teenager is a toddler in a grown-up body; they are both risk takers with similar fears.

INITIAL ASSESSMENT

The challenge of triaging pediatric patients stems from several key factors:

- Anatomical differences
- Developmental considerations
- Anxiety and fear in both the patient and parent or caregiver

Fast Facts

- Children often present with signs and symptoms that are vague and nonspecific, and they have the potential to suddenly decompensate.
- *All* children must be assessed upon arrival; failure to do a quick visual observation of neonates, infants, and young children, can lead to devastating consequences. Consider the infant who arrives bundled in a carrier and covered with a blanket with parents who state he or she "has a cold and is sleeping." Let's further suppose that, for whatever reason, there is a lapse of 20 minutes or longer prior to an assessment by a nurse. Imagine the horror of removing the blanket and finding a blue, apneic baby in the carrier.
- *All* children must be assessed upon arrival!

A rapid initial observational assessment tool is the Pediatric Assessment Triangle (PAT; Chameides, Sampson, Schexnayder, & Hazinski, 2011). There are three components to the PAT:

1. General *appearance*: Level of consciousness, muscle tone, spontaneous movements, look/gaze, and cry
2. Work of *breathing*: Retractions (e.g., sternal, intercostal, supraclavicular), nasal flaring, positioning (e.g., tripod, head bobbing), audible airway sounds
3. *Circulation* to skin: Skin color (e.g., gray, mottled, cyanotic, pale)

The PAT provides the nurse with a general impression of the physiological status of the patient and assists the experienced nurse to appropriately prioritize patients. This assessment can be performed in any order and should not take longer than 60 seconds to perform. An abnormal assessment should prompt the nurse to facilitate immediate placement of the patient in an appropriate treatment area with the necessary resources at the stretcher-side. (For additional information on the PAT, see tinyurl.com/q394pzh [Auerbach, 2016].)

The PAT is followed by:

- Primary assessment (airway, breathing, circulation, and disability)
- Secondary assessment (chief complaint and focused examination along with vital signs)

Although different throughput processes guide where and by whom this assessment takes place, the components do not change. This assessment process is completed by the head-to-toe assessment.

"See, I Am a Kid"

Part of the triage assessment process involves obtaining subjective data. Subjective data include anything the caregiver or patient tells you, often referred to as the history—both past history and history of current illness or injury. The mnemonic ***C-I-AM-PEDS*** (*"see, I am a kid"*) was developed to ensure the collection of relevant data when assessing pediatric patients (Emergency Nurses Association, 2012a). Its use encourages a systematic approach to obtaining information, making it less likely that important details will be missed (Emergency Nurses Association, 2012a):

C	Chief complaint
I	Immunizations, isolation
A	Allergies
M	Medications
P	Past medical history, parent's impression
E	Events surrounding illness or injury
D	Diet, diapers
S	Symptoms

Fast Facts

- Infants are at increased risk for dehydration. Inquiring with the caregiver the amount of diaper changes (e.g., wet or diarrhea) in the past 24 hours is important.
- Best practice when weighing a child up to 3 years of age is to weigh without clothing.
- Questions to help determine amount of vomitus in a young child include:
  - Could you wipe the vomitus off the child with a diaper or rag?
  - Was a change of clothes needed for the infant or caregiver?
  - If vomit was on a bed, sheet, or floor, how big of a circle did it make?
  - Does vomiting occur after every feeding?
  - Did it look like what was just eaten, or was it curdled?
  - What color was the vomit?
  - Was the vomit projected away from the child?

A Word About Vital Signs

Any pediatric patient who will not be immediately placed in the treatment area should have vital signs assessed. Remember that "normal" vital signs do not always reflect the physiological stability of the child due to the pediatric patient's ability to compensate. *Always* assess the patient to get a complete picture. Although numerous references provide vital sign parameters for various age groups, it is interesting to note the lack of consistency in the literature as to what defines the limits of "normal" ranges (Hohenhaus, Travers, & Mecham, 2008). Posting normal vital sign ranges at triage provides for easy reference and is highly recommended.

A plethora of literature acknowledging the multifaceted vulnerability of pediatric patients exists; however, nowhere is this more evident than in the realm of medication errors. Therefore, all pediatric patients should be weighed in kilograms (using a kilogram-only scale). The weight should be recorded in an easily identifiable area of the medical record (American Academy of Pediatrics, Committee on Pediatric Emergency Medicine, American College of Emergency Physicians, Pediatric Committee, & Emergency Nurses Association Pediatric Committee, 2009; Emergency Nurses Association, 2012b).

Fast Facts

- A pulse oximetry reading is not necessary to determine acute respiratory distress. Assess work of breathing (e.g., seesaw respirations, use of accessory muscles, and nasal flaring). A child may be able to maintain a pulse oximetry measurement greater than 90% and still be in severe distress. Remember that *respiratory compromise is the source of most pediatric arrests.*
- Normal pediatric blood pressure is calculated using the following equation:

    $$70 + (2 \times \text{age in years})$$

- A change in blood pressure in a child is a late finding.

Caution: Be on the Lookout!

Numerous symptoms should alert the astute triage nurse to a critically ill or injured child. See tinyurl.com/lp8q949 for specific presentations applicable to the primary assessment of airway, breathing, circulation, disability, and exposure (ABCDE). The Emergency Nursing Pediatric Course covers this content in greater detail. In addition to the presentations discussed in this chapter, anytime a child is reported by the parent or caregiver as behaving in a way that is unlike his or her normal behavior, pay careful attention.

Fast Facts

Use distraction techniques appropriate to the developmental stage of the child to accomplish your assessments. For example, an infant aged 6 to 12 months may be distracted by a brightly colored toy attached to your stethoscope while a 2-year-old may be more distracted by blowing bubbles with a wand.

PEDIATRIC PRESENTATIONS: TRIAGE PERILS

Apparent Life-Threatening Event

The presentation of an apparent life-threatening event is often assigned a lower acuity level at triage because the infant looks "just fine" upon arrival. Do not be fooled; *any* infant with a reported episode of apnea, color change, or change in muscle tone, accompanied by choking or gagging, is a high-acuity patient. Anticipate the immediate need for continuous cardiac and pulse oximetry monitoring. Parents often describe an episode in which they believed that the infant had died.

Bronchiolitis

A very common condition in young children and infants, bronchiolitis represents a constellation of infections, the most common of which is respiratory syncytial virus (RSV). RSV occurs most often in winter and early spring, especially in very young or premature infants, and can be life-threatening. Be prepared for frequent nasal suctioning, especially in obligate nose breathers. Moving them out of triage as soon as you are able is a good idea.

Child Abuse

Knowledge of developmental stages is important in order to detect when a child is potentially being abused or neglected. Be very attuned to injuries that are inconsistent with developmental stages or history. For example, it is extremely unlikely that a 6-month-old fell and sustained a femur fracture while walking. On the other hand, bruising to a 2-year-old's shins is common as children this age often fall as they toddle about. A full discussion of child abuse and neglect is beyond the scope of this chapter, but always remember you *must* report suspected child abuse to the authorities. Do not assume that another provider or social worker is reporting suspected abuse. As nurses, we are expected to report our concerns as well since we are mandated reporters!

Fast Facts

> Drooling that is inappropriate for the age of the patient is a "red flag" that should get your immediate attention.
> Any neonate (0–28 days) with a fever of 100.4°F (38°C) or greater is a high-risk presentation.
> If a baby is excessively crying without an apparent reason, check the fingers, toes, and penis for a hair tourniquet.

Croup

Croup is a very common childhood illness in which upper airway obstruction occurs as a result of inflammation and swelling. By the time stridor is present, significant airway swelling has occurred. Anticipate the need for humidified blow-by oxygen, dexamethasone, and nebulized racemic epinephrine.

Fever

Fever accompanies a wide range of illnesses, from minor to life-threatening. When assessing children, remember that fever, or lack thereof, does not necessarily indicate severity of illness. A child can be hypothermic, normothermic, or hyperthermic and be critically ill.

Foreign Body Aspiration/Obstruction

Young children like to put anything and everything into their mouths. Foreign body aspiration is *most common* in children younger than age 3 years. If a young child presents with sudden onset of respiratory distress without a known precipitating event, think possible foreign body aspiration or obstruction.

Intussusception

The classic presentation for intussusception (telescoping of the bowel into another segment of bowel) is intermittent episodes of sudden acute abdominal pain during which the child typically flexes the knees (94%). The child may also vomit after the pain has begun. The classic presentation includes "currant jelly" stool with bloody mucus approximately 25% of the time. This condition usually occurs between 3 months and 5 years of age, peaking between 3 months and 1 year of age. In between episodes the child may appear nondistressed. A barium enema is often both diagnostic and therapeutic! Surgery, however, may be required if the barium enema is unsuccessful. Keep the patient NPO.

Nursemaid's Elbow

With nursemaid's elbow, subluxation of the radial head occurs after forceful jerking of the arm (e.g., being pulled by the arm). The child holds the arm in a position of comfort and typically refuses to use it. Think mechanism of injury with this one!

Pyloric Stenosis

Forceful projectile vomiting after feeding is a classic symptom of pyloric stenosis. Although it can occur anywhere from birth to approximately 5 months, the most common age is 3 to 4 weeks. This type of vomiting is due to a congenital obstruction at the pyloric sphincter. The vomiting may or may not be accompanied by a palpable mass the size of an olive above the umbilicus as well as visible wavelike peristalsis across the abdomen. Symptoms include continued hunger after feeding, poor weight gain, and few bowel movements. Keep the patient nothing by mouth (NPO). Beware! These infants may present already demonstrating signs of dehydration, shock, and malnutrition!

References

American Academy of Pediatrics, Committee on Pediatric Emergency Medicine, American College of Emergency Physicians, Pediatric Committee, & Emergency Nurses Association Pediatric Committee. (2009). Joint policy statement—Guidelines for care of children in the emergency department. *Pediatrics, 124*(4), 1233–1243. doi:10.1542/peds.2009-1807

Auerbach, M. (2016). Pediatric resuscitation technique. In D. J. Nimavat (Ed.), *Medscape*. Retrieved from http://tinyurl.com/q394pzh

Chameides, L., Sampson, R. A., Schexnayder, S. M., & Hazinski M. F. (Eds.). (2011). *Pediatric advanced life support provider manual*. Dallas, TX: American Heart Association.

Emergency Nurses Association. (2012a). *Emergency nursing pediatric course: Provider manual* (4th ed.). Des Plaines, IL: Author.

Emergency Nurses Association. (2012b). *Position statement: Weighing pediatric patients in kilograms*. Retrieved from https://tinyurl.com/y9pa87au; http://www.ena.org/SiteCollectionDocuments/Position%20Statements/WeighingPedsPtsinKG.pdf

Hohenhaus, S., Travers, D., & Mecham, N. (2008). Pediatric triage: A review of emergency education literature. *Journal of Emergency Nursing, 34*(4), 308–313. doi:10.1016/j.jen.2007.06.022

Newman, B., & Newman, P. (2014). *Development through life: A psychosocial approach* (12th ed.). Independence, KY: Cengage.

31

Older Adult Triage

Anna Sivo Montejano

Today there are more people than ever before over the age of 65 years. By the year 2050, projections are that one out of five Americans will be older than 65 (Touhy & Jett, 2015). As a result of this expanding population of older Americans, many facilities see increased numbers of older adult patients who are seeking medical care for their complaints. Special consideration should be given to this population because they may arrive with atypical presentations that can be overlooked in the triage arena, putting them at risk for deterioration or even death. Gathering information relevant to the older adult patient's complaint can be challenging because of possible sensory deficits or physical limitations. A keen eye and patience will allow the nurse to gather the information needed to assign an accurate acuity level and facilitate the most appropriate disposition following triage. This chapter provides communication and examination tips along with types of abuse that this specific population is exposed to.

Upon conclusion of this chapter, you will be able to:

1. State three physical changes that occur to the older adult.
2. State three types of violence against the older adult population.
3. Explain an atypical presentation in an older adult.

OLDER ADULT ASSESSMENT

As people become older, physiological changes occur throughout the body, including respiratory, cardiovascular, and musculoskeletal systems. This is an ongoing process as we age. When performing a physical assessment, an awareness of these physiological changes is important because the changes put the patient at risk for additional problems (e.g., dehydration).

Some Physical Changes

- Respiratory system
  - Stiffening of the chest wall
  - Decrease in chest wall compliance and functioning alveoli and cilia
- Cardiac system
  - Decrease in cardiac output, stroke volume, and heart rate in response to stress
  - Stiffening of the arteries (elastin loss)
- Integumentary system
  - Decreased subcutaneous fat
  - Increased capillary fragility (easily bruised)

Some Emotional Changes

- Depression
  - Loss of significant other (e.g., living alone)
  - Loss of friends
- Caregiver role fatigue
  - When caring for an elderly spouse (e.g., an 80-year-old wife with a physically or mentally disabled 83-year-old husband may be "on call" as the primary caretaker 24/7)

Potential Risks

- Malnutrition
- Dehydration
- Cardiovascular disease
  - Remains the leading cause of death in adults older than age 85 (Lewis et al., 2017)
- Medication interaction (polypharmacy)

Critical thinking and application of older adult knowledge can decrease the patient's risk for a poor outcome by leading to early initiation of needed interventions.

> **Fast Facts**
>
> - Older patients often delay seeking help for their problems, alerting the nurse to *consider* a higher acuity level when they do present with health complaints.
> - If you need to remove an article of clothing while assessing the older patient (e.g., to take a blood pressure reading), complete the task as quickly as possible to minimize his or her discomfort (e.g., feeling cold).

COMMUNICATING WITH AN OLDER ADULT PATIENT

Assessing the older adult population relies on the nurse's critical thinking and decision-making skills. Often the older adult patients will not seek help until it is absolutely necessary or their loved ones force them to be evaluated. Many older adults are independent and self-sufficient and fear having that independence taken away. When communicating with these individuals, be aware of their feelings and express compassion about their concerns. The triage process typically takes more time when caring for the older adult; be patient. Rushing older adult patients often prolongs the process as they may become easily flustered.

Reasons for Communication Delays

- Possible short-term memory loss
  - Recalling the specifics for the visit may offer challenges
- Their perception is that they will be seen quickly and then released
- Many questions asked by multiple people causes:
  - Frustration
  - Irritation
  - Misunderstanding (especially if English is not their first language)
- A high priority is for them to return home quickly to care for a loved one or pet

Tips for Effective Communication With the Older Adult Population

- Speak slowly and clearly.
- Do not ask too many questions at once.
- If the patient is hard of hearing, speak in a lower tone of voice.
- Provide reassurance.

- Do not refer to the patient as "honey," "sweetie," or in similar terms:
  - These words can be interpreted as disrespectful or condescending.
- Keep your promises.
- Be honest.
- Recognize that there may be a delay in obtaining information in triage:
  - Some patients may tell you more than you need to know, including details of a vacation or about a family member who had similar symptoms years ago.
  - Patients may have brought numerous medications for the nurse to sort through.
- Allow the patient to make choices, even if small ones:
  - Where do you want me to put your eyeglasses?
- Ask for permission if you need to assist in removing an article of clothing.

Older adult patients can be set in their ways and particular about how their personal possessions are handled or put away. Be respectful and conscious of their concerns. Certain personal items may be expensive or sentimental. A healthcare provider who attempts to remove or displace these items can cause anxiety to the patient.

Examples of items of concern to the older adult:

- Keys
- Medications
- Medical cards
- Dentures
- Eyeglasses
- Purse or wallet

EXAMINATION TIPS

The following simple examination tips can facilitate the assessment, making the process a relatively easy experience instead of an anxiety-provoking one (for the patient) and lengthy (for the nurse or medical provider).

Suggestions for the Older Adult Examination in Triage

- Only expose areas being examined; older adult patients get cold easily.
- Provide warm blankets if able.
- Assist the patient with removal of clothing if needed; ask for permission to do so.
- Ask closed-ended questions:
  - Questions that require only yes or no answers limit the discussion of unnecessary information.

POLYPHARMACY

Polypharmacy, a situation in which a patient is taking multiple medications, often occurs in the older adult population. It can cause adverse drug reactions that may go unnoticed by the treating medical provider or lead to additional medications being prescribed to treat the patient's new complaint. However, these additional medications can, in turn, cause further drug-related problems.

Potentially inappropriate medications commonly used in the older adult:

- Clonidine
- Cyclobenzaprine
- Diazepam
- Diphenhydramine
- Hydroxyzine
- Ketorolac
- Meperidine
- Nifedipine
- Promethazine
- Propoxyphene (Donatelli & Somes, 2013)

The triage nurse must be on alert for older adult patients who present to the triage area with complaints such as confusion or dizziness. The nurse's first thought may be that the patient is experiencing a neurological issue, but a complete medication history, including over-the-counter medications, and a heightened awareness of drug reactions may lead to a different conclusion.

ATYPICAL PRESENTATION

An atypical presentation, simply defined, is one that does not manifest with expected symptoms and signs. Atypical presentations can result in missed diagnoses, and this issue is of particular concern in older adult patients because their complaints are often vague or nonspecific. For example, an acute myocardial infarction is often misdiagnosed or overlooked because the older adult patient arrives with a complaint of general weakness, epigastric discomfort, or confusion. As healthcare providers, we are listening for classic descriptions like chest pain, nausea, or diaphoresis. The presence of risk factors (e.g., diabetes) should increase the nurse's awareness that the patient may be in danger. Recognizing and appropriately intervening can make a difference in the patient's outcome.

ELDER ABUSE

Older adult patients are at risk for abuse due to their vulnerability and dependence on others for help. Unfortunately, all too often a trusted individual is the abuser.

Types of abuse:

- Physical
- Neglect
- Psychological
- Sexual
- Financial
- Abandonment

Be aware of this worldwide phenomenon and take time to listen to your patients. If you receive any information that raises your suspicion that elder abuse may be occurring, follow through and notify appropriate personnel. Your actions may contribute to stopping the abuse. Recognition of an abusive situation while a patient is in your care may be the patient's only chance for intervention.

Fast Facts

Elder abuse goes largely unreported. The key to identifying abuse is to use all of your senses and to recognize that this problem occurs in all settings and at all societal levels.

CULTURAL COMPETENCE

Today's nurses will most likely deliver care to patients who are of a different culture, reinforcing the need for culturally competent care. It is expected that by the year 2050, the groups currently designated as minorities in the United States will become the majority (Touhy & Jett, 2015). Cultural competence includes not only an awareness of our own personal values and beliefs but also those of other individuals in our community.

In certain cultures, pain is not expressed outwardly. If a patient presents to triage with a complaint of chest pain but appears calm and without pain, the nurse may interpret this symptom as "no big deal." This interpretation may erroneously lead us to believe that the patient is stable because he or she is not exhibiting signs of pain or distress. As a result, the patient may be assigned a lower-than-warranted acuity level, leading to an inappropriate disposition.

Fast Facts

If a nurse is unaware of cultural differences and approaches patients as if everyone responds the same to any given situation, an inaccurate acuity designation may be assigned, resulting in a negative outcome.

References

Donatelli, N. S., & Somes, J. (2013). Beers list: What's NOT on "tap" for the older adult? *Journal of Emergency Nursing, 39*(5), 491–494. doi:10.1016/j.jen.2013.07.008

Lewis, S. L., Bucher, L., Heitkemper, M. M., Harding, M. M., Kwong, J., & Roberts, D. (2017). *Medical-surgical nursing: Assessment and management of clinical problems* (10th ed.). St. Louis, MO: Elsevier.

Touhy, T. A., & Jett, K. (2015). *Ebersole & Hess' toward healthy aging: Human needs and nursing response* (9th ed.). St. Louis, MO: Elsevier.

32

Pain Management at Triage

Reneé Semonin Holleran

Pain remains one of the primary complaints that causes patients to seek medical care. Pain can be either acute or chronic. Overall, there has been a significant increase in the number of patients who present to the ED with a pain complaint. Reasons include lack of funds to consult a pain management specialist; work hours that do not allow them to be seen by a primary care provider; trying to deal with the pain on their own and being encouraged or told to use the ED for care by their primary care providers. Issues related to the opioid crisis have also presented unique challenges to pain management in the ED.

Upon completion of this chapter, you will be able to:

1. Define acute and chronic pain.
2. List three triage questions related to pain assessment.
3. List three methods to manage pain in the ED.

ACUTE AND CHRONIC PAIN

Pain has been described and defined in numerous ways. In 1994, the International Association for the Study of Pain (2017) defined pain as "an unpleasant sensory and emotional experience associated with actual or potential tissue damage or described in terms of such damage."

Acute Pain

Acute pain is a protective mechanism that occurs when nociceptors, or sensory neurons, present in areas of the body, including the skin and the viscera, respond to the damaging stimuli by sending pain signals to the spinal cord and the brain. Damaging stimuli may include heat or cold, mechanical trauma, illness (e.g., cholecystitis or appendicitis), or procedural interventions (e.g., surgical procedure). The pain should resolve when the cause of the pain has been managed or removed and/or the damaged tissue has healed.

Chronic Pain

Chronic pain is described as persistent noncancer pain that lasts more than 3 to 6 months. Causes of chronic pain are not well understood but may be related to such problems as chronic inflammation. In addition, risk factors for the development of chronic pain include maladaptive pain coping behaviors and psychiatric illnesses such as depression and posttraumatic stress disorder (PTSD). Chronic pain can significantly impact the quality of a person's life.

MANAGING PAIN AT TRIAGE

Each facility should have a policy that describes how pain should be assessed, documented, and managed in the triage area.

Assessing Pain

A good history, including asking PQRST questions (discussed in Chapter 10), can help the triage nurse understand the circumstances surrounding the patient's pain and then intervene appropriately. Further insight into a patient's pain can be obtained by asking additional questions, which include:

- If the pain is chronic, what is different about it now?
- For patients with a history of chronic pain, what is a tolerable level of pain for them?

Fast Facts

Asking questions that help you understand how the pain interferes with the patient's ability to function (e.g., work, sleep, eat, or care for themselves) can provide great insight into the severity of the person's pain. In addition, observing the posture of the patient (e.g., hunched over, not able to lie flat) can provide added invaluable information.

Treating Pain at Triage

Pain management interventions that might be performed in triage include:

- Splinting
- Application of ice or heat
- Distraction
- Medication administration (e.g., acetaminophen, ibuprofen, intranasal analgesia)
- Therapeutic touch
- Essential oils
- Repositioning

RED FLAG FINDINGS THAT MAY INDICATE RISK FOR DRUG OVERDOSE

Some individuals are at a greater risk for drug overdose and include those with the following:

- Reported history of addiction or medication diversion
- History of opioid overdose
- Injection or inhalation of opioid preparations
- Using or stealing other patient's pain medications
- Use of illicit medications, such as methamphetamines or heroin
- Medication use, such as benzodiazepines with opioids

Fast Facts

In the United States in 2016, 66.4% of drug overdose–related deaths involved opioids that were either illicit, prescribed, or a combination of both (Seth, Rudd, Noonan, & Haegerich, 2018). These staggering statistics have led to new regulations for medical providers in when and how much opioid medication to prescribe. Utilizing alternative forms of pain control are more important than ever. Consider asking the patient if he or she has taken too much of an opioid pain medication or has been exposed to opioid medication belonging to another individual, and anticipate the potential need to administer nasal naloxone 4% if indicated.

References

International Association for the Study of Pain. (2017). IASP terminology. Retrieved from http://www.iasp-pain.org/Education/Content.aspx?Item Number=1698

Seth, P., Rudd, R., Noonan, R., & Haegerich, T. M. (2018). Quantifying the epidemic of prescription opioid overdose deaths. *American Journal of Public Health, 108*(4), 500–502. doi:10.2105/AJPH.2017.304265

33

Patient and Staff Safety

Anna Sivo Montejano

> Violence seems to be everywhere in our society. News media and newspapers are saturated with stories of violent acts, and you may have experienced violence personally or professionally yourself. As a triage nurse, you are highly vulnerable to both verbal and physical forms of violence. Since the triage area is often set apart from the rest of the department, isolation and seclusion are real concerns. The patient volume of the facility may dictate the number of resources available at triage. For example, a rural ED may have only one triage nurse who also functions as the charge nurse and a staff nurse, whereas higher census facilities may have multiple staff at triage. No matter the size of the facility, one common theme is that the occurrence of violence is inevitable.

Upon conclusion of this chapter, you will be able to:

1. Identify what causes a patient to become agitated, which can lead to violence.
2. State two types of violence.
3. Identify three ways to provide a safe environment.

TYPES OF VIOLENCE

- *Verbal abuse* is one form, which consists of yelling, swearing, threatening, accusing, intimidating, making demands, or simply raising one's voice.

- *Physical abuse* is the attacking of an individual or threatening the person physically; it includes physically throwing objects, from small items, such as a pencil, to large items such as a wheelchair; at times there is biting, spitting, grabbing, or punching—the list goes on.

POTENTIAL FOR VIOLENCE

What makes a person violent? Often we wonder why anyone would be violent toward us. After all, we are here to help patients recover from their illness or injury. Why do some people begin yelling before we are given a chance to show them how nice we are? Why do they become angry when we are not able to take them to a bed immediately upon their arrival? Do patients not realize our resources are limited and that their visit is just one of the nearly 120 million ED visits that occur annually in the United States? Recognizing that some individuals have characteristics that increase their chances of becoming violent while others are influenced by situational or environmental factors is important.

Qualities of a Potentially Violent Patient or Visitor

- Intimidating
- Threatening
- Brisk pace
- Mumbling
- Loud speech; demanding
- Using profanity
- Rapid speech
- Entering another individual's personal space
- Throwing objects
- Under the influence of drugs or alcohol

Situational Reasons for Agitation

- *Miscommunication.* Imagine an elderly parent with complaints of fever and vomiting. The daughter calls the physician, who tells her to go directly to the ED, where "there will be a bed waiting for your mother." When the family arrives at the ED, the triage nurse informs them that there is no bed available and that the ED has not received a call from the physician. This initial miscommunication, increases the chance that the daughter (or another accompanying family member) may exhibit frustration or agitation toward the triage nurse.
- *Crowded waiting room (WR).* A patient presents for medical care and finds the WR packed. The line of people wanting to be seen flows from the front desk, out the door, and into the hall. People occupy all the WR chairs, wheelchairs obstruct the staff's

ability to walk, and some of those waiting are even sprawled on the floor. This sight alone can be overwhelming, even without the noises and smells experienced upon entering the WR. The patient quickly realizes that the chances of being seen in a short period of time are extremely slim. In this situation, the many sights, sounds, and smells of the WR, and the likely lengthy time it will take to be seen, can combine to increase his or her anxiety, resulting in agitation and the potential for violence.

- *Ambulance arrival.* A patient is transported to the hospital by ambulance only to be sent to the WR. Envision the patient's arrival: The gurney is brought out to triage and the patient is unloaded. As a triage nurse, this does not faze you in the least. This practice is common in facilities that handle large numbers of patients. Those with low-acuity level complaints are often taken to triage. However, this can be extremely frustrating to the patient, who may have expected to be placed in a bed upon arrival. The patient may respond by using abusive language and may become agitated. Be aware this situation may result in a potential for violence. Be safe!
- *Insurance.* Some patients who have insurance assume they will be seen before those who are uninsured.
  - Example: A male patient with insurance arrives at the ED with a complaint of a laceration to the finger after opening a box with a box cutter. Five minutes later an uninsured, homeless man arrives with complaints of ischemic chest pain. The triage nurse takes the homeless patient with chest pain to the treatment area first. Visibly upset, the first patient approaches the triage nurse and, leaning forward into the nurse's personal space, loudly verbalizes that because he has insurance and arrived first, he should be given priority.
- *Patients comparing themselves to others with the same complaint.* Occasionally two patients arrive with seemingly identical complaints, but the person who arrives later is taken for evaluation before the patient who arrived first.
  - Example: Patient A arrives with her significant other, complaining of a migraine. Your comprehensive assessment shows normal vital signs, no neurological deficits, no past medical history, and no reported allergies. The patient has self-diagnosed herself with a migraine. Patient B arrives also complaining of a migraine. After completing the comprehensive triage assessment, the nurse is concerned because of the patient's history of breast cancer and her report that this headache "feels different" than her usual migraines. Patient B is brought for evaluation first. Patient A,

or her significant other, may become angry because of their perception of the situation. The triage nurse should be aware that agitation may ensue.

Ways in Which ED Staff Play a Role in Increased Patient/Visitor Agitation

- Restricting the patient's choice
  - Example: Not allowing a patient to drink or eat but failing to explain why may agitate the person.
- Restricting visitation
- Not keeping one's promise
  - Example: Visitors would like to see their mother, who is a patient in the ED. They are told someone will come and get them in "a minute." Thirty minutes later they are still waiting.
- Denying a comfort measure
  - Example: A patient requests a warm blanket or the visitor asks for a cup of water and is denied without an explanation.
- Communicating incongruently (e.g., verbal communication does not match nonverbal communication)
- Failing to provide information or reassessment or both
  - Example: A patient has been waiting 3 hours to be seen by a provider. No update or information is provided about the wait time, nor is a reassessment completed by the triage nurse. This lack of information or compassion may result in increased agitation.

Fast Facts

- The key to decreasing violence in the triage area is *prevention*. Assessing the risks for agitation, including behavior, environment, and the staff's role, can help in de-escalating a situation before it progresses to violence.
- Staff education in management of aggressive behavior (MOAB) is a must. Additional information can be obtained at www.moabtraining.com/main.php. In addition, the Emergency Nurses Association provides a toolkit on workplace violence at www.ena.org/docs/default-source/resource-library/practice-resources/toolkits/workplaceviolencetoolkit.pdf?sfvrsn=6785bc04_30 and an online workplace violence course at www.ena.org/practice-resources/workplace-violence.

BEHAVIORAL HEALTH PATIENTS

Psychiatric conditions can be a factor in agitation leading to violence. Many patients arrive at triage with some level of psychosocial emergency. Those with a history of psychiatric illness may have trouble processing external stimuli and are often less able to handle the environment of the ED. Additionally, they may not understand why they do not receive immediate care. Some aspects of their illness make it difficult to think rationally, which may increase the tendency to react with violence. Triage nurses must be able to differentiate patients who are restless, irritable, or having hallucinations (e.g., auditory, visual), and those who may be a danger to themselves or others, and respond in a caring and sensitive manner.

ALCOHOL AND SUBSTANCE ABUSE

Alcohol, drugs, and illicit substances that are used separately or in combination can create a volatile situation when an impaired patient is brought to triage. The triage nurse must have a heightened awareness of the risks in this situation to stay safe and keep the patient safe. When interacting with an individual who is under the influence of alcohol or drugs, the triage nurse must pay close attention to the person's verbal responses. The patient may be loud, use foul language, and may encroach on the nurse's personal space, causing the nurse to feel uncomfortable.

Imagine a crowded WR in which a patient under the influence of alcohol starts yelling loudly about his disapproval of the wait time. This situation sparks a patient with an unknown illegal drug in his system to begin yelling at the first patient who is under the influence. Neither patient is capable of rational responses, limiting how far they will go because they are not attuned to their surroundings or the consequences of their behavior. After the verbal altercation, both individuals stand up and approach one another. If no one intervenes, a potentially violent situation may occur. The triage nurse needs to recognize what is occurring, call for assistance to defuse the situation, and strive to provide a safe environment for everyone.

SECURITY

Security is utilized in different ways within medical facilities worldwide and includes:

- Weapon-carrying officers employed by or contracted with the facility
- Security guards trained in de-escalation techniques (these guards do not carry weapons)

- Officers or security guards who may be regularly stationed in the area or nearby; at times a phone call is necessary to alert these guards to the need for additional assistance
- Metal detectors or wands used upon entry to the facility to ensure the safety of patients and staff

Smaller facilities, because of lack of resources, may rely on their employees to act as security. Whatever the case may be in your facility, the importance of having well-trained security or other staff available to work with the medical team is critical to minimize the chance of a violent situation occurring.

INCREASING SAFETY IN THE TRIAGE AREA

Measures to increase safety in the triage area are important to ensure that a secure environment is provided for patients, visitors, and staff. Some changes are costly while others have a minimal effect on the budget.

Changes to Make an Area Safe

- Increase lighting in dark areas.
- Always have an exit route plan.
- Provide all visitors with a name tag stating the room they are visiting; this practice discourages visitors from wandering the department and encourages staff to play an active role in recognizing who belongs where.
- Enclose the triage area (e.g., with bullet-resistant glass).
- Install hidden panic buttons that staff can press to alert security or deliver an overhead announcement.
- Install closed-circuit cameras or video recording.
- Provide security attendants when needed.
- Provide training for staff in management of aggressive behavior (MOAB) and interpersonal communication.

Keeping the Triage Nurse and Others Safe

The triage nurse's ability to communicate effectively plays a strong role in his or her ability to keep patients and visitors from becoming anxious or confrontational and in reducing the likelihood that these heightened emotional responses will escalate to agitation or ultimately explode into violence.

Techniques to Keep Safe

- Active listening can help alleviate a patient's or visitor's anxiety and convey a feeling of reassurance. By listening to an individual's concerns, the nurse also demonstrates that he or she cares for the individual's well-being.

- Be aware of your nonverbal communication; these behaviors and cues express 80% of what you are communicating.
  - Leaning forward shows interest in what the patient is saying.
  - Standing or sitting at the same level as the patient or visitor helps create a connection between you and the individual.
  - Placing your hands by your side rather than folded across the chest expresses a feeling of openness.
  - Using *I* statements, such as "I understand what you are saying," provides a reassuring and nonaccusatory response to the individual.
  - Using eye contact with your head at an angle rather than straight on appears less confrontational.
  - Speaking in a normal tone even if the patient is yelling can help diffuse the situation.
- Keep your promise; if you say you will be back in a minute, follow through.
- Keep patients updated; lack of information can increase anxiety and frustration.

Fast Facts

Being honest and truthful conveys a feeling of caring in an environment that is dynamic and sometimes chaotic.

34

Case Studies in Triage Nursing

Anna Sivo Montejano and Lynn Sayre Visser

Everybody has a story, scenario, or case study they can share from their experiences working in various clinical settings. Articles, books, and magazines can increase a person's knowledge regarding disease processes, peculiar lab results, and unusual imaging findings. However, real-life experiences are what most people never forget. No need to memorize or think of a mnemonic, your remembrance is enough. Cases like these make you think, "Wow, I am happy I learned that!" The following case studies could occur anywhere and in any department. This chapter provides scenarios that will raise your awareness of some high-risk, low-frequency situations.

Upon conclusion in this chapter, you will be able to:

1. List one important precursor to a catastrophic event in an infant.
2. State why you should never disclose to outside sources that an inmate is located within your department.
3. Identify one observation that may lead you to suspect domestic violence.

CASE STUDIES

Newborn Not Eating

A neonate was brought to triage by her parents with a report of poor feeding and excessive sleeping. The triage nurse's first thought was

"A newborn sleeping a lot is completely normal!" The new parents appeared anxious. Reassurance was given and they decided to go home, feeling silly for overreacting. The following day, the baby continued to eat poorly and appeared listless, so the worried parents returned to the ED. Upon arrival, the triage nurse removed the blanket covering the baby carrier and discovered the neonate in respiratory arrest. The ED staff successfully resuscitated the baby. The final diagnosis was sepsis. ***Remember:*** Sometimes symptoms described by parents or caregivers may be vague or seem of minimal concern, but often. Catastrophic events are vague in nature. Pay attention to comments such as "poor feeding" or "something is just not right" and always remember to look under the blanket. Do not let guard down; a life is at stake!

Diarrhea

An unkempt homeless female patient arrived via ambulance, complaining of diarrhea and abdominal pain. No rooms were available within the department. Triage did not seem like a good option because of her intermittent loud cries and her inability to sit in a chair so she was placed on a hallway gurney. She was immediately assessed with the usual questions for a female in her 40s with abdominal pain. The patient's responses raised no immediate concerns for the nurse. Throughout the next hour the patient repeatedly and rapidly climbed off the gurney and leaned forward while walking toward the bathroom. When questioned, such as on the date of her outbursts, the patient stated she was having diarrhea and did not feel well. As the nurses scurried about caring for their high-acuity patient assignment, one nurse noticed that the patient's cries of pain seemed almost rhythmic. A few more questions were asked about her last menstrual cycle, the possibility of pregnancy, vaginal bleeding, and so on. The patient adamantly stated there was no chance of pregnancy because she was currently on her period and had not "done it in years!" Just as the patient began to scream, the nurse lifted up the sheet. The head of a lifeless, blue-faced baby was protruding between the patient's legs. Quickly the staff intervened, successfully resuscitating the baby. ***Remember:*** Never let your guard down, because the chance to save a life may be just around the corner.

Inmate

Caring for inmates in our ED was common. They came in handcuffed, escorted by police, the sheriff, or a correctional officer, and as long as they were handcuffed and an escort was present, the staff typically felt safe. Then one day the ED phone rang and the person on the line asked for a patient by name. Not thinking much about it, the nurse said, "Oh yes, he is here. Do you want to talk to him?"

The person hung up. The nurse thought, "That was kind of rude!" He approached the officer to let him know that someone had called asking for this inmate. The officer's face went pale. At first the nurse did not realize what he had done. He assumed the caller was another officer or someone from the jail. Before he knew it, the officer was making multiple phone calls and requesting that the patient be admitted to the hospital as soon as possible. Only then did the nurse realize the dangerous situation he had created for each individual within the department. When an inmate is no longer in a secured area with locked gates, officers, and continuous surveillance, the inmate becomes a prime target to either escape with the help of his friends or be eliminated with the help of his enemies. **Remember:** One must never disclose to outside sources that an inmate is in the facility. Sharing this information can potentially put the officers, staff, visitors, and inmate at risk.

Suicidal Patient

A patient presented to triage stating he had a cut on his arm. He appeared unfazed by the injury and spoke in a monotone voice. The patient was asked how the injury occurred, and he simply stated "I cut myself." The nurse proceeded to ask, "What did you cut yourself with?" He pulled a scalpel out of his pocket, and placed it on the counter. To the nurse's surprise, the scalpel was from the facility's ED. The patient was immediately escorted to a private area for further questioning, and the nurse inquired if he had anything else with which he could use to harm himself. He calmly removed a knife with an 8 inch (20 cm) blade from his pocket. No further injury occurred to the patient and everyone remained safe within the ED. **Remember:** By asking appropriate questions and remaining calm, the triage nurse can play a big role in safe outcomes.

Feeling Funny

Sometimes patients describe symptoms that do not seem to make sense or easily fit into any acuity category, but intuition leads us to make the right decision. A 60-year-old woman arrived to triage with vague complaints of not feeling well, ringing in her ears, and a funny feeling in her chest. She had an irregular heartbeat, 76 bpm, blood pressure 122/70, respiratory rate 18 breaths per minute, and she was afebrile. Her only past medical history was atrial fibrillation. The nurse identified the patient as a high-risk presentation and acted accordingly, placing the patient in a treatment room. Initially the patient was stable, but after 1.5 hours there was much commotion in her room. When asked what the ruckus was about, the bedside nurse showed the triage nurse the patient's cardiac rhythm strip that showed *4-second pauses*. The "funny feeling in her chest" now made a lot of sense.

Remember: Connecting the dots between the patient's chief complaint and signs and symptoms is a critical role of the triage nurse. Always pay attention to the subtle clues.

Foot Pain

A woman in her 40s approached the triage check-in. A man with two children in a stroller stood behind her as the nurse inquired about the reason for seeking care. "I hurt my foot," she replied. The nurse looked down to see the woman wearing flip-flops. The top of her left foot was discolored and twice the size of the right foot. When the triage nurse asked what had happened, the woman reported, "I tripped." The nurse looked more closely at the foot but could not imagine how a trip-and-fall injury could cause the degree of swelling and discoloration that had occurred. She noticed that the man stayed close to the woman throughout the triage assessment and often spoke for her. Feeling uneasy with the story, the triage nurse realized she needed a moment alone with the patient to ask further questions. When a technician came to take the woman for a foot x-ray, the triage nurse knew this was her opportunity to further inquire about the injury, so she escorted the patient to radiology. In a concerned tone, the nurse asked the patient if she had been assaulted, which the patient adamantly denied. The nurse gently expressed concern that the injury looked like a crush injury from someone or something stomping on her foot. "You do not need to tell me what happened, but I need you to know that I'm concerned for you," said the nurse. During the short encounter, the triage nurse provided the patient with an orthopedic business card. The card was not intended for orthopedic follow-up but rather had the number for the organization Women Escaping a Violent Environment (WEAVE). At triage the patient's story does not always match the clinical findings. When this occurs, going the extra mile to ask further questions is a must. *Remember:* Intimate partner violence is a real concern. Your actions could potentially help or save the life of a person at risk.

Fast Facts

Despite busy shifts in triage, always stop long enough to make eye contact with each patient, *listen* to their concerns, *look* at their area of complaint, and incorporate *touch* into your assessment. *Compassionate care* and *compassionate actions* go a long way with patients and visitors.

VII

Disaster Situations in Triage Nursing

35

Emergency Management: A Triage Nurse's Guide for When Disaster Strikes

Erik Angle

Disasters can occur as an internal disaster (e.g., fires, utility failures, chemical spills, cyberterrorism, or active shooters) or an external disaster (e.g., severe weather events, pandemics, active shooters/threat, or terrorist incidents). The success in disaster management depends on rapid recognition and response to the event. The goal for healthcare facilities is to treat the medical conditions of the patients in need of care. Disaster incidents can cause a surge in patients to the facility and staff must be prepared to activate the facility's emergency response plans. Incoming patients are evaluated with multicasualty incident (MCI) triage and the command center is established to meet the needs of the events. Emergency management has distinct cycles or phases, which include mitigation, preparedness, response, and recovery. This chapter covers the phases of emergency management and keys for each of them.

Upon conclusion of this chapter, you will be able to:

1. Identify the four phases of emergency management and provide examples for each.
2. Identify the "zones" in a hazardous materials incident.
3. Identify levels of disaster or MCI triage.

PHASES OF EMERGENCY MANAGEMENT

The four phases of emergency management are mitigation, preparedness, response, and recovery. Each of these stages will be discussed in the content that follows. This information is not all encompassing but should give you a foundation if faced with a situation requiring an emergency response.

Mitigation

Mitigation Defined: Activities that prevent a disaster from occurring, reduce the likelihood of the occurrence, or reduce the damaging effects of unavoidable hazards.

Mitigation Goal: Reduce the probability or the impact of the disaster to the facility.

Mitigation Examples: An example of mitigation is a hazard vulnerability assessment (HVA). Facilities assess the probability of disasters that place the facility at risk based on historical data (e.g., risks that have actually occurred based on facility location and history). The HVA may include multidisciplinary hospital personnel as well as community partners (e.g., healthcare emergency coalition members, emergency medical service [EMS], fire, law enforcement). Another example of mitigation would be the installed backup emergency generators that can provide ongoing power for the facility when power fails.

Preparedness

Preparedness Defined: Well-developed plans for what to do, where to go, or who to call for help before an event occurs. These actions will improve the chances of successfully dealing with an emergency or disaster.

Preparedness Goal: The preparedness goal for hospitals is to achieve a state of readiness and response to a disaster and remain functional to treat medical conditions of those in their communities. During disaster incidents, there is still a goal to treat those within the community and the surge of injured victims can increase the critical nature of the incident.

Preparedness Examples:
- Maintaining a current and effective emergency operations plan (EOP).
  - Adopting and practicing policies and procedures for major emergencies.
  - Predesignation and identification of temporary/emergency equipment sites (e.g., designated locations for surge capacity tents, decontamination resources, hospital spaces to be used for patient surge care) to address the identified risks.
  - Permanent improvements or upgrades (e.g., permanent decontamination facility, electronic locks for door security,

communications improvements, information technology [IT] infrastructure improvements for cyber threats) to address the identified risks.
- Training to address the identified risks (e.g., stop-the-bleed training, evacuation triage).
- Hospital incident command system (HICS) assignments. Providing training for those roles is vital for readiness and continuity of operations, including off-shift events and replacement staff.

Fast Facts

Disaster drills and exercises should be developed based on identified risks and emergency plans. Coordination with law enforcement, fire departments, EMS, and other community partners should occur. Developing these relationships and participating in drills *prior* to an incident occurring is critical.

Response

Response Defined: The actions taken to save lives and minimize damage to property.

Response Goals: Putting the preparedness plans into action while maintaining staff, patient, and visitor safety. Response success depends on how prepared the facility is and how it responds in a crisis.

Response Examples: Response levels can be tailored (e.g., limited or alert vs. full or activate, staff recall, implement access control) to the incident types, to the facility, and to the community the facility serves. An MCI may temporarily strain hospital resources as the number of casualties exceeds bed capacity, available supplies, and staffing.

- **MCI/Trauma Incidents:**
  - Motor vehicle or transportation incidents cause a significant amount of trauma-related disaster incidents, often without notice and with many casualties
  - Active shooter and active violence (e.g., nonfirearm weapons, knives, vehicles)
  - Natural disaster incidents (e.g., earthquakes, wildfires, flooding, hurricanes, mudslides)
- **MCI/Medical Incidents:**
  - Medical MCIs occur when patient care surges from a nontrauma situation and overwhelms the hospital and local healthcare delivery system (e.g., pandemic illness, food poisoning).
  - Medical MCIs often involve multiple victims in a single geographic region, may gradually occur over time, and then have a drastic influx of ill patients presenting for care.

- When medical MCIs occur, one must consider the possibility of intentional or accidental poisoning (e.g., food, air, water, mailed packages).
- Proper protective equipment is essential during disaster events to protect caregivers. Resource management is essential; notify the facility supply department and local public health department early in the planning stages to manage these and other critical resources.
- Resource allocation must be discussed early in the event, especially in pandemic or highly infectious disease response. The public health department along with hospital personnel should have protocols in place with trigger points for "austere care conditions" to help make these extremely difficult decisions.

- **MCI/Hazardous Material Incidents:**
  - Hazardous materials (hazmat) pose a unique and complicated challenge to receiving healthcare facilities that are there to treat patients and provide care rapidly. Contaminated patients pose a significant threat to the staff, other patients, and the facility.
  - The triage nurse must be able to recognize contaminated patients and know how to activate the emergency response if necessary.
  - The contamination risk and patient influx could come from internal or external incidents, such as an accidental release of toxic chemicals (e.g., train derailment, motor vehicle collision, industrial accident) or an intentional terrorist attack (e.g., nerve agent release, radiological dispersal device). Hazmat incidents could also involve burns, traumatic injuries, or even radiation exposure dependent upon the nature of the incident.
  - Victims may vary widely in their severity of symptoms, from the simply "worried well" to the critically injured.
  - Toxidromes are the clinical signs and symptoms related to chemical exposure. There are varying toxidromes for the chemicals that patients may be exposed to. Organophosphate or nerve agent poisoning causes distinct toxidrome symptoms known with the mnemonics following:
    - SLUDGEM (Salivation, Lacrimation, Urination, Defecation, Gastrointestinal Distress, Emesis, Miosis/Muscle Fasciculation)
    - DUMBBELLS (Diarrhea, Urination, Miosis/Muscle Weakness, Bronchospasm, Bradycardia, Emesis, Lacrimation, Lethargy, Salivation)
  - Healthcare facilities receiving patients must prepare for the potential need for mass decontamination. Perimeters help define contaminated areas and assist to create control zones where the

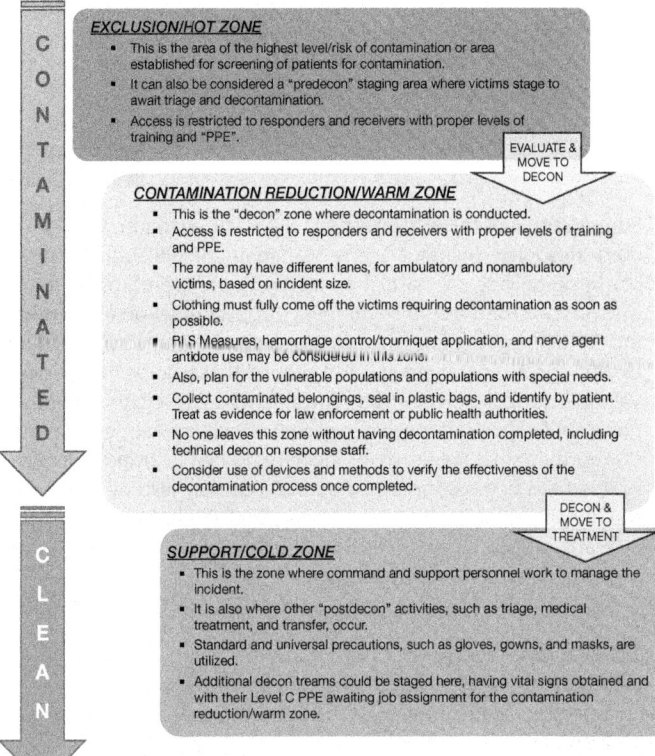

Figure 35.1 Decontamination Control Zones
BLS, basic life support; PPE, personnel protective equipment.

contamination can be contained. These zones would be for any form of potential contamination that is dangerous to life, property, and environment (e.g., chemical, biological, and radiological/nuclear materials). Recommended areas (control zones) and patient flow for mass decontamination include exclusion/hot zone, contamination reduction/warm zone, and support/cold zone. Additional information is available in Figure 35.1.

- Decontamination areas could be built-in decontamination systems and showers and decontamination trailers/tents, and some may simply have a hose and a pop-up pool.
- Once the decontamination is completed, personnel assigned to the decontamination team must go through suit and

equipment decontamination (technical decontamination) and then remove the protective decontamination suits they were wearing. Once these suits are removed, vital signs are taken for the caregiver and rest and hydration should occur.

> **Fast Facts**
>
> Something new to MCI/Hazardous Materials Incidents are The Primary Response Incident Scene Management (PRISM) guidelines. These guidelines are part of an international program developed on science-based response for mass decontamination of chemical-incident casualties. Endorsed by the United States Department of Health and Human Services and others, these guidelines provide valuable tools to ensure that all patients exposed to potentially hazardous chemicals receive the most effective treatment possible during the initial stages of an incident. PRISM is primarily utilized by the field first-responder personnel but may also be utilized by the hospital-based first-receiver personnel. PRISM information and operational guides are available at https://www.medicalcountermeasures.gov/barda/cbrn/prism

- **MCI/Disaster Triage:**
  - An MCI may temporarily strain hospital and healthcare resources as the number of casualties exceeds bed capacity, resources, and staffing. The sudden surge of victims can present major challenges. Altering the methods of triage to a standardized color-coded MCI triage system would assist with the surge.
  - The goal of triage is to *rapidly* sort patients according to their urgency while keeping in mind resources needed and the likeliness of survival.
  - There are many varying MCI triage methods available, and it is important to know what your facility and region uses. The more common systems used in the United States are simple triage and rapid treatment (START) triage, pediatric JumpSTART triage, and sort, assess, lifesaving interventions, triage and/or transport (SALT) triage. More information on these topics is available at https://chemm.nlm.nih.gov/triage.htm. Whatever method of disaster triage is used, a color-coded system based on respiration, perfusion, and mentation is used. Modifications have been developed for EMS, fire, and hospitals on how to handle casualties in a nuclear/radiological disaster incident. Figure 35.2 was developed as a national all-hazard mass casualty system and is the recommended national standard for all patients/victims.

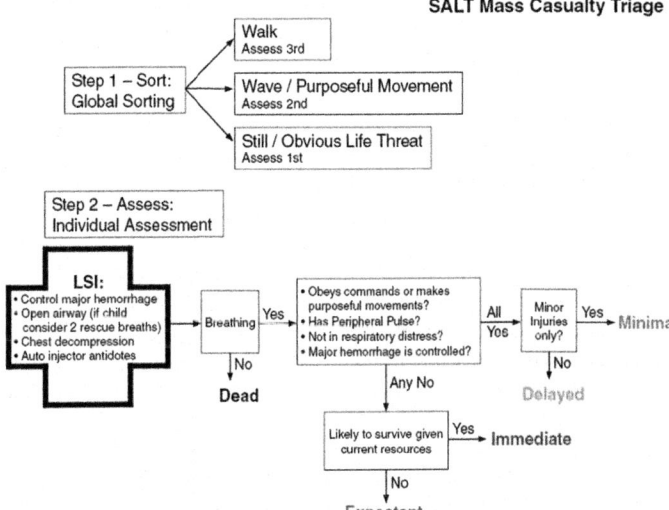

Figure 35.2 SALT Mass Casualty Triage
LSI, lifesaving interventions; SALT, sort, assess, lifesaving interventions, triage and/or transport.
Source: American College of Surgeons Committee on Trauma, American Trauma Society, National Association of EMS Physicians, National Disaster Life Support Education Consortium, and State and Territorial Injury Prevention Directors Association. *Disaster Med Public Health Prep.* 2008 Dec;2(4):245–6, © Society for Disaster Medicine and Public Health, Inc. 2008.

Fast Facts

A sample disaster triage tag, courtesy of the New Jersey Department of Health, is located in Appendix E. Many areas use a similar type of triage tag for MCIs. Being familiar with the triage tag utilized in your area before a disaster strikes is crucial to efficient MCI triage.

Recovery

Recovery Defined: The process of returning to preincident status. This process is initiated as objectives are met and resources no longer needed are released, returned, or replaced and the hospital returns to the normal business practice of providing patient care.

Recovery Goal: Safe and efficient return to normal daily hospital operations or the continuation of operations based on the "new normal" (e.g., providing care in mobile field hospital while damage repaired or facility rebuilt). Identification of lessons learned and assigning corrective actions that would mitigate future impacts of disasters.

Recovery Examples: Both hospital and staff/personal recovery needs to take place.

Hospital Recovery:

- If the hospital emergency plans were activated for a threat that was minimal in nature (e.g., a small internal fire), demobilization and recovery may take only a few minutes.
    - For larger disasters (e.g., hurricane, wildfire, mass shootings), the recovery phase may last days or even longer.
    - Recovery operations include equipment rehabilitation, restocking, documentation, financial accounting, restoration of electronic healthcare data, restoring backups, and rescheduling of postponed procedures.
    - Improvised patient care areas (e.g., surge capacity tents, conference rooms) would return to their prior state.
    - Conduct after-action review(s) and develop a corrective action plan with staff assignments for carrying out those actions. Recognize the strengths when the hospital succeeded and identify opportunities to improve future responses.

Staff/Personal Recovery:

- Personal recovery for the hospital staff. Depending on the incident (e.g., wildfire, hurricanes), staff may have lost personal property (e.g., homes, vehicles) or even lost loved ones.
- After a large-scale natural disaster, staff members returning home may deal with issues that are both physically and emotionally challenging.
- Mental health is a great concern for staff and responders during a disaster. Staff may require a critical incident stress debrief/psychological first aid debrief.
- Psychological debriefing should be offered for staff and volunteers.
- Signs of disaster-related stress may include difficulty sleeping, limited attention span, headaches/stomach problems, disorientation/confusion, depression, feelings of guilt, sadness, and feelings of hopelessness.

Reference

U.S. Department of Health and Human Services. (2017). *SALT mass casualty triage algorithm*. Retrieved from https://chemm.nlm.nih.gov/salttriage.htm

36

Active Shooter or Active Violence

Erik Angle

Active shooter and active violence incidents are a threat that can happen anywhere, any time, and can happen without warning. Many of these incidents are revenge in nature but can also be due to ideological extremism. The assailants routinely have specific targets but may hit innocent victims or "targets of opportunity" who are around them. These incidents are usually random and predatory in nature. They evolve quickly, and a rapid response is critical to save lives. This chapter covers some incident definitions, how to prepare yourself for an active shooter situation, and critical stress management after the incident.

Upon conclusion of this chapter, you will be able to:

- State three ways in which you can prepare yourself in an active shooter situation.
- Identify incident-predicting warning signs.
- List immediate response steps and recovery.

PREPARING THE FACILITY AND YOURSELF

A number of steps should be taken to adequately prepare for an active shooter or active violence situation prior to such an event. Preparation may include:

- Complete a facility annual risk assessment to evaluate risks and provide physical and operational measures to prevent these incidents from occurring.

- Active shooter or active violence training should be provided as part of the workplace violence prevention training (e.g., management of aggressive behavior training) and should also be offered to personnel in standalone courses.
- Stop-the-bleed training should be incorporated into the required basic life support (BLS) training and should be required for all staff members (including security services).
- Obtain wall-mounted or bagged trauma kits for staff response, as well as bystander response, for hemorrhage control.
- Educational training, drills, and exercises should be offered, with all staff members encouraged to participate. Provide a full-scale exercise in which simulated victims are involved and actual real-time simulated incident response occurs.
- Regardless of the type of education or exercise, planning, coordination, and invitations should be extended to law enforcement, fire departments, emergency medical service (EMS), and other community partners (e.g., Red Cross, Amateur Emergency Radio Services, Public Health) and even to federal agencies (e.g., Federal Bureau of Investigation [FBI]) when applicable.

Fast Facts

- Developing relationships with outside agencies such as law enforcement, fire department personnel, other EMS personnel, and so on *before* an incident occurs is critical.
- According to a recent study released by the FBI (n.d.), of the 250 active shooter incidents that occurred in the United States from 2000 to 2017, only 5 of those incidents occurred at hospitals. In these incidents, 3 people were killed and 12 were wounded. Of the shooters, 4 committed suicide and 1 was killed by law enforcement.

SITUATIONAL AWARENESS—WARNING SIGNS

As a triage nurse, **situational awareness** and recognizing potential threats of active shooter or active violence risk are crucial. If these signs are recognized, security and/or your human resources department (if behaviors or actions come from staff members) should be notified. Early recognition of behavioral warning signs in patients, visitors, and even staff or former staff can save lives.

Behavioral Warning Signs

Behavioral warning signs may include:
- Violent fantasy content and increased comments on violence. This may include increased comments on violence, stories they wrote, or manifestos depicting violence.

- Inappropriate fascination with weapons, especially those designed to kill, such as machine guns, semiautomatic pistols, snub nose revolvers, stilettos, bayonets, daggers, brass knuckles, special ammunition, and explosives
- Pseudocommando mentality
- Boasting and practicing fighting skills for no identified reason.
- Loner or recluse who is isolated and socially withdrawn.
- Unexplained increase in absenteeism and/or vague physical complaints
- Homicidal ideation and violent contempt for others
- Paranoia and comments of being singled out, abused, or persecuted
- Pathological fixation on a person or an extremist cause

Informational Leakage Warning Signs and Statistics

- Leakage can be defined as the communication to a third party of an intent to do harm to a target through an attack.
- Leakage statistics:
  - In adult active shooters, 51% had leaked intent to third parties before an attack.
  - In active shooters 17 and younger, 88% leaked information prior to attack.
  - In an FBI (n.d.) study of school shooters, all (100%) engaged in some sort of preattack leakage.

Fast Facts

Incident Statistics of the Shooters/Attackers:

- Forty-three percent of the time, the shooting had ended before law enforcement arrived.
- Ninety-seven percent were male perpetrators and most often between the ages of 21 and 50.
- Ninety-eight percent were single perpetrators; 90% committed suicide after attack.
- Seventy-five percent bring multiple weapons; 35% extensively planned for the attack.

Incident Statistics of the Victims/Targets:

- No specific age, gender, race, religion, or nationality
- Intent to create the highest casualty rate before being confronted by police
- Seventy-nine percent of active shooters demonstrated they were acting with a grievance/grudge of some kind toward a specific target or targets

SITUATIONAL AWARENESS—WEAPON CONCEALMENT

Recognizing an individual who may be concealing a weapon, whether it is a firearm or other weapon, and responding and reporting this observation is vital to saving lives.

- **Self-Security Check:** The assailant with the weapon wants to ensure that the weapon is still there. The most common areas to conceal a weapon are the waistband and pockets.
- **Quick Adjustments:** Some weapons, especially firearms, can be difficult to keep in place due to their uneven distribution of their weight. Individuals may make quick movements or adjustments of the hands to keep in contact with their weapons.
- **Body Blading:** When assailants find it necessary to walk through a crowd, they do not want the weapon felt or recognized by anyone else. They may blade or take an oblique stance and shift their upper body away as they move or stand still to avoid a face-to-face encounter and shift their body to keep the weapon out of line of sight.
- **Weapon Palming:** Assailants, especially those who are concealing an edged weapon, may keep the weapon hidden along their arm or leg to keep it from being seen. They may keep their hands in their pockets and not remove them when asked to do so.
- **Conspicuous Clothes:** Those attempting to conceal weapons may be wearing clothes that appear unseasonable, odd, mismatched, or out of place:
    - Clothes do not suit the weather/season, such as a bulky jacket closed in hot weather to conceal the weapon.
    - Bulges or sagging seen with their clothes. A holstered gun may appear as a lump when the arms are extended or lifted or the individual bends at the waist.
    - Jacket does not fit evenly to conceal the weapon in the pocket.

INCIDENT RESPONSE

The risk of an active shooter or active violence incident is *higher in the community* than within the hospital itself.

Attack Occurs in the Community

When an attack happens within the community (not within your facility), you should do the following:

- Assume the role as assigned in the hospital's emergency operations plan (EOP) and prepare for incoming mass casualties.
- Recognize that there is the potential that the hospital could be a secondary target.

Attack Occurs Within the Hospital/Healthcare Facility

Active shooter or active violence incidents in a healthcare setting present unique challenges, such as a large vulnerable patient population and hazardous materials. There are special challenges such as with firearms and MRI machines (these machines contain large magnets that can cause accidental discharge of a weapon or may physically remove the weapon from the hands of law enforcement). To be prepared for an attack within your facility, you should know the following:

- How to initiate your facility policy for active shooter or active violence incident response.
- Be aware of the standardized hospital emergency code for active shooter or active violence incident. Codes may vary from color-based codes (e.g., Code Silver, Code Black) to plain language–based codes (e.g., "Security Threat: Active Shooter") or may even be a hybrid of both (e.g., "Code Silver, active shooter" with the location mentioned and other plain language instructions that follow). It is important to know what your facility uses before you need it.

Attack Occurs Within Your Department/Unit

If an active shooter or active violence incident occurs in your department/unit, do the following:

- Remain calm! Your thought process must switch from daily operations to survival mode, which is *run, hide, and fight.*
- **Run,** *evacuate the immediate area,* and warn others as able:
  - If safe to do so, remove patients from hallways or take them with you.
  - Close patient doors and instruct them to turn off the lights and be quiet. If patients are mobile, instruct them to potentially hide in their bathrooms and lock the bathroom door.
  - Leave personal belongings behind but *take your cell phone* if you have it on you. Be sure to *silence your cell phone* but do not turn it off.
  - Do not attempt to move or treat wounded people unless you have the time, the training, and it is safe to do so.
  - Do not activate the fire alarm.
  - Do not stay behind if others are not willing to go.
- **Hide,** *if running and evacuation is not an option.* Hide in a securable location, such as rooms with lockable doors (e.g., bathrooms, lounges, medication rooms). Lock, secure, and barricade doors by any means (e.g., using furniture, cabinets, bed, and belt). It is important to know which way the door will swing to do this successfully.
- **Fight**, if your life and the lives of others are at *immediate risk*. You need to *fight your own fear* and fight the attacker because fear can be your worst enemy in these incidents:

- Instinct and nature will work against you. As your heart rate increases, your self-control will decrease.
- There are two subconscious body functions that can be consciously controlled, eyeblinking and breathing. Four deep four-count breaths and consciously slowing down your blinking may slow your heart rate, lower your stress level, and bring your body back under some degree of control.
- If it is decided to *fight the attacker*, try to *coordinate with others* for maximum impact. Use objects in your immediate environment as weapons (e.g., fire extinguishers, laptops, trauma shears, and hot coffee). Commit to your actions to *fight like lives depends on it, because they do.*

Attack Happens Outside Your Department/Unit

If the active shooter or active violence incident occurs outside your department/unit, you should do the following:

- Avoid the announced area of threat.
- Close and secure doors to your department, such as main doors, hallway doors, and even doors to the patient rooms, and stand by for further instructions.
- *Do not* let visitors, patients, and other staff members leave the area or walk the halls. If you are concerned that the threat may impact the patients in the waiting room/lobby, plan to calmly evacuate those patients to a secondary more secure location.
- Staff members with medical training may be requested to assist with victim evacuation and basic first aid if the scene is safe.
- Remain in "lockdown" mode until you hear "All clear" declared.

Prepare for Law Enforcement Response

The initial responding law enforcement team has a singular purpose of *stopping the attacker* and will not assist victims. When they arrive, do the following:

- Remain calm and follow their instructions.
- Expect that you may be yelled at and forcibly placed to the ground as a physical protective measure.
- Do not argue or fight with the police; they will consider you a threat and act accordingly.
- Anticipate that you will have weapons pointed at you by law enforcement.
- Avoid pointing, running, or screaming at them.
- Keep your hands raised, open, and away from your body.
- Ask for permission before reaching for objects under desks, clothing, and so on.

STOP THE BLEED

Research and history have indicated that the active risk at most incidents is over before first responders arrive on scene, or shortly thereafter. Definitive medical care *may be delayed* until the shooter is stopped and hospital personnel may be the initial first rescuers. *Remember:* The victims may be the shooter, patient, visitor, your coworker, your best friend, or even your family.

- **Identify "life-threatening" bleeding, for example:**
  - Blood that is pooling on the ground
  - Clothing and/or bandages that are soaked with blood
  - Bleeding in a victim who is now confused or unconscious
- **If you do not have a trauma or first aid kit:**
  - Open the clothing by tearing or cutting over the bleeding wound. While lifesaving measures always come first, attempt to keep bullet or knife holes in the clothing intact to preserve evidence.
  - Wipe away any pooled blood to visualize injury.
  - Apply direct pressure on the wound. Cover the wound with a clean cloth and apply pressure by pushing directly on it with both hands.
  - Take any clean cloth (e.g., a shirt) and cover the wound.
  - If the wound is large and deep, try to "stuff" the cloth down into the wound.
  - Even if you as a rescuer have to improvise, avoid using paper products, such as paper towels or toilet paper, to stop the bleeding.
  - Apply continuous firm pressure with both hands directly on top of the bleeding wound until relieved by medical responders.
- **If you *do* have a trauma or first aid kit:**
  - Follow the steps listed under "If you do not have a trauma or first aid kit" but use the supplies in your kit, such as bleeding control gauze (preferred), plain gauze, or clean cloth, to control bleeding.
  - Stuff the wound with packing, especially if there is bleeding from an arm, leg, neck, shoulder, or groin.
- **CAT (combat application tourniquet) or similar tourniquet *is available* and there is life-threatening bleeding from an arm or leg:**
  - Open the clothing by tearing or cutting over the bleeding wound. While lifesaving measures always come first, attempt to keep bullet or knife holes in the clothing intact to preserve evidence.
  - Wipe away any pooled blood to visualize the injury.

- Wrap the tourniquet around the bleeding arm or leg about 2 to 3 inches (5–7.5 cm) above the bleeding site (***do not*** place the tourniquet onto a joint; place above the joint if necessary).
- Pull the free end of the tourniquet to make it as tight as possible and secure the free end onto Velcro.
- Twist the windlass until bleeding stops and secure the windlass rod in the holder. A tourniquet ***will cause*** some pain but this is necessary to stop life-threatening bleeding.
- Note the time the tourniquet was applied.
- ***If the bleeding does not stop*** with the single initial tourniquet, you may ***apply a second tourniquet*** 2 to 4 in. (5–10 cm) above the first tourniquet. Follow the same procedure as previously discussed for the second tourniquet. *Do not release these tourniquets until arrival at a trauma facility.*

CRITICAL INCIDENT STRESS MANAGEMENT

- These incidents may occur with little to no warning and cause powerful emotional reactions in people who are exposed, especially children. The choices you make may stay with you forever.
- Recognize signs of critical incident stress, such as difficulty sleeping, limited attention span, headaches/stomach problems, disorientation or confusion, depression, feelings of guilt, sadness, and feelings of hopelessness. Acknowledging these feelings, focusing on your strengths, and knowing when and how to accept help can assist you in recovery.
- Psychological first aid and employee assistance programs can assist with incident stress debriefing and counseling.
- Recognize that if the assailant survives, the criminal trial may cause a prolonged impact on your emotions and the emotions of others directly involved.
- Recognize the 1-year anniversary of the incident and the emotional difficulty it may have on you and the emotions of others directly involved.

Reference

Federal Bureau of Investigation (FBI). (n.d.). *Quick look: 250 active shooter incidents in the United States from 2000 to 2017*. Retrieved from https://www.fbi.gov/about/partnerships/office-of-partner-engagement/active-shooter-incidents-graphics

Abbreviations

ABC	airway, breathing, and circulation
ABCDE	airway, breathing, circulation, disability, and exposure
ACLS	Advanced Cardiac Life Support
ACS	acute coronary syndrome
ADLS	Advanced Disaster Life Support
AMA	against medical advice
AMI	acute myocardial infarction
ASA	acetylsalicylic acid
ATP	advanced triage protocol
ATS	Australasian Triage Scale
AVPU	alert, verbal, pain, unresponsive
BDLS	Basic Disaster Life Support
BLS	Basic Life Support
BM	bowel movement
BNP	B-type natriuretic peptide
bpm	beats per minute
C&S	culture and sensitivity
CAT	combat application tourniquet
CBC	complete blood count
C-diff	Clostridium difficile
CEN	Certified Emergency Nurse
cm	centimeters
CMP	complete metabolic panel
CMS	Centers for Medicare and Medicaid Services
COBRA	Consolidated Omnibus Budget Reconciliation Act of 1985
COPD	chronic obstructive pulmonary disease
CPEN	Certified Pediatric Emergency Nurse

CPK	creatine phosphokinase
CPR	cardiopulmonary resuscitation
CSE	commercial sexual exploitation
CST	child sex trafficking
CT	computed tomography
CTA	computed tomography angiography
CTAS	Canadian Triage Acuity Scale
CTP	computed tomography perfusion
CXR	chest x-ray
DKA	diabetic ketoacidosis
DO	doctor of osteopathy
DTaP	diphtheria, tetanus, and pertussis
DUMBBELLS	diarrhea, urination, miosis/muscle weakness, bronchospasm, bradycardia, emesis, lacrimation, lethargy, salivation
ECG	electrocardiogram
ED	emergency department
EMC	emergency medical condition
EMR	electronic medical record
EMS	emergency medical service
EMTALA	Emergency Medical Treatment and Active Labor Act
ENA	Emergency Nurses Association
ENPC	Emergency Nurse Pediatric Course
EOP	emergency operations plan
ER	emergency room
ESI	Emergency Severity Index
ETAT	Emergency Triage Assessment and Treatment
FBI	Federal Bureau of Investigation
ft	feet
GCS	Glasgow Coma Scale
GENE	Geriatric Emergency Nurse Education
GI	gastrointestinal
GPS	global positioning system
HCG	human chorionic gonadotropin
Hct	hematocrit
HELLP	hemolysis, elevated liver enzyme levels, and low platelet levels
Hgb	hemoglobin
HHS	hyperosmolar hyperglycemic state
HICS	hospital incident command system
HIPAA	Health Insurance Portability and Accountability Act
HIV	human immunodeficiency virus
HVA	hazard vulnerability assessment
I&Os	intake and outputs
ICD	implantable cardioverter defibrillator

ICU	intensive care unit
in.	inch
INR	international normalized ratio
IPV	intimate partner violence
IV	intravenous
kph	kilometers per hour
L	liter
LBTC	left before treatment complete
LGBTQ	lesbian, gay, bisexual, transgender, questioning/queer
LGI	lower gastrointestinal
LOQ	line of questioning
LOS	length of stay
LPMSE	left prior to the medical screening exam
LVAD	left ventricular assist device
LWBS	left without being seen
LWT	left without treatment
m	meters
MAP	mean arterial pressure
MCI	multicasualty incident
MD	medical doctor
mg/dL	milligrams per deciliter
MI	myocardial infarction
mL	milliliter
mmHg	millimeter of mercury
mmol/L	millimoles per liter
MMR	measles, mumps, and rubella
MOAB	management of aggressive behavior
mph	miles per hour
MRI	magnetic resonance imaging
MSE	medical screening exam
MTS	Manchester Triage System
NG	nasogastric
NIHSS	National Institutes of Health Stroke Scale
NP	nurse practitioner
NPO	nothing by mouth
NSAID	nonsteroidal anti-inflammatory drug
PA	physician assistant
PALS	Pediatric Advanced Life Support
PAT	Pediatric Assessment Triangle
PCV	pneumococcal vaccine
pH	potential hydrogen
PHI	personal health information
PID	pelvic inflammatory disease
PMH	past medical history

PPE	personnel protective equipment
PQRST	provokes and palliates; quality; region and radiation; severity and symptoms; timing and temporal relations
PT	prothrombin time
PTSD	posttraumatic stress disorder
PTT	partial thromboplastin time
QMP	qualified medical person
Rh	rhesus
RICE	rest, ice, compression, and elevation
RMC	retail medical clinic
RN	registered nurse
RSV	respiratory syncytial virus
r-tPA	recombinant tissue plasminogen activator
RUQ	right upper quadrant
SALT	sort, assess, lifesaving interventions, triage and/or transport
SARS	severe acute respiratory syndrome
SBP	systolic blood pressure
SIRS	systemic inflammatory response syndrome
SLUDGEM	salivation, lacrimation, urination, defecation, gastrointestinal distress, emesis, miosis/muscle fasciculation
SOAP	subjective, objective, assessment, plan
ST	sex trafficking
START	simple triage and rapid treatment
STD	sexually transmitted disease
STEMI	ST-segment elevation myocardial infarction
TCRN	Trauma Certified Registered Nurse
TDD	telecommunication device for the deaf
TIA	transient ischemic attack
TNCC	Trauma Nursing Core Course
TTD	text-telephone device
UA	urinalysis
UCC	urgent care center
UGI	upper gastrointestinal
US	ultrasound
VAD	ventricular assist device
WBC	white blood cell
WEAVE	Women Escaping a Violent Environment
WR	waiting room
°C	degrees Celsius
°F	degrees Fahrenheit
<	less than
>	greater than
%	percent

Appendix A: Resources

OTHER BOOKS BY THE AUTHORS

- Visser, L., & Montejano, A. (2018). *Rapid access guide for triage and emergency nurses: Chief complaints with high risk presentations.* New York, NY: Springer Publishing.

FORMALIZED TRIAGE EDUCATION

- Emergency Nurses Association has online triage education modules available at www.ena.org
- Triage First, Inc., offers both online and live triage education opportunities at www.triagefirst.com
- Health Resources Unlimited, Inc., has online and live education accessible at www.hru.net
- Emergency Triage Assessment and Treatment (ETAT) course
- 2011 Guidelines for Field Triage of Injured Patients Course for EMS Professionals at www.cdc.gov/mmwr/preview/mmwrhtml/rr6101a1.htm

WEBSITES

Additional triage knowledge can be gained from the following websites:

- Emergency Nurses Association Triage Position Statement at www.ena.org/docs/default-source/resource-library/practice-resources/position-statements/triagequalificationscompetency.pdf

- *The Emergency Severity Index*, fourth edition, provides access to a free download at www.ahrq.gov/professionals/systems/hospital/esi/index.html
- The American College of Obstetricians and Gynecologists offers information on Hospital-Based Triage of Obstetric Patients at www.acog.org/Clinical-Guidance-and-Publications/Committee-Opinions/Committee-on-Obstetric-Practice/Hospital-Based-Triage-of-Obstetric-Patients
- Canadian Triage Acuity Scale (CTAS) resource links and information about mobile device application purchases is available at ctas-phctas.ca
- Emergency Triage Assessment and Treatment (ETAT) course manual for participants is available at www.who.int/maternal_child_adolescent/documents/9241546875/en
- Australian Government Department of Health and Ageing Emergency Triage Education Kit is available at www.health.gov.au/internet/main/publishing.nsf/content/casemix-ed-triage+review+fact+sheet+documents

Appendix B: Triage Competency Validation Form

Orientee Name:	Preceptor Name/Initials:	
Employee No.:	Date:	
Criteria	Criteria Observed (O) or Verbalized (V)	Preceptor Initials
Performs a rapid triage assessment to obtain the patient's chief complaint		
Utilizes the chief complaint to drive questions to identify life-threatening situations		
Identifies an impairment in the A-B-C-D-E assessment		
Acts appropriately on an impairment in the A-B-C-D-E assessment		
Identifies vital sign abnormalities for pediatric, adult, and older adult patients		
Lists potential worst-case scenarios related to the chief complaint		
Utilizes the chief complaint to ask appropriate medical history questions		
Obtains chief complaint subjective and objective triage data		
Drives the triage interview with open- and closed-ended questions		
Identifies factors that may impact the interview (e.g., disability, language barrier)		
Documents the patient's chief complaint and objective and subjective data		

(continued)

(continued)

Criteria	Criteria Observed (O) or Verbalized (V)	Preceptor Initials
Initiates appropriate advanced triage protocols when indicated		
Identifies patient allergies before administering medication		
Maintains patient privacy		
Identifies the patient requiring isolation		
Isolates potentially infectious patients per facility policy		
Communicates pertinent data to the medical provider when applicable		
Performs comprehensive triage assessment when appropriate and per policies		
Identifies surge capacity and requests additional personnel resources appropriately		
Accurately prioritizes multiple waiting patients		
Utilizes triage alerts (e.g., trauma, stroke) per policies		

Appendix C: Sample Triage Education and Competency Plan

Requirements Before Orienting to Triage	■ Practice as an RN for a minimum of ___ month(s)* ■ Practice in the facility for a minimum of ___ months
Education	■ Successful completion of foundational triage education ■ Education related to critical thinking skills ■ Self-assessment tool with triage scenarios ■ Remediation plan (if applicable)
Competency Validation	■ Retrospective chart review of ____% of triage records each shift ■ Team feedback (including providers') related to effective professional communication skills while in triage role ■ Identification of ability to apply critical thinking skills related to red flag recognition at triage (chart reviews and observation) ■ Identification of any mistriages or unacceptable/unprofessional behaviors or practices in the role of the triage nurse (chart reviews and observation) ■ Direct observation with preceptor for ___ shifts

Ongoing Triage Competency Evaluation	■ Determine frequency of the following (may be annual, biannual, or based on changes in practice standards)
	  ▪ Triage update education
	  ▪ Clinical updates on "red flags," "near misses," or new patient demographic risk categories
	  ▪ Retrospective triage chart review (self-review and/or peer review); identify number of records and patient types to be reviewed with a specific frequency
	  ▪ Team feedback (including providers) related to effective professional communication skills while in the triage role

*The Emergency Nurses Association currently recommends a minimum of 1 year of experience as an RN before orienting to triage. The most up-to-date recommendations can be found at www.ena.org.
RN, registered nurse.

Appendix D: Sample Triage Retrospective Chart Review Audit Form

ADULT CHEST PAIN

Select five adult patient records with a chief complaint of chest pain, excluding any trauma-related patients. Check the box reflective of what you documented at the time of the actual triage.

Note whether the following was documented in the triage nurse notes:

Record #	Onset of Pain Sudden, Gradual, etc.	Other Symptoms	Quality of Pain	Triage Level	Meet Triage Criteria?*	Comments**
	YES ❑ NO ❑	YES ❑ NO ❑	YES ❑ NO ❑			
	YES ❑ NO ❑	YES ❑ NO ❑	YES ❑ NO ❑			
	YES ❑ NO ❑	YES ❑ NO ❑	YES ❑ NO ❑			
	YES ❑ NO ❑	YES ❑ NO ❑	YES ❑ NO ❑			
	YES ❑ NO ❑	YES ❑ NO ❑	YES ❑ NO ❑			
	YES ❑ NO ❑	YES ❑ NO ❑	YES ❑ NO ❑			
	YES ❑ NO ❑	YES ❑ NO ❑	YES ❑ NO ❑			
	YES ❑ NO ❑	YES ❑ NO ❑	YES ❑ NO ❑			
	YES ❑ NO ❑	YES ❑ NO ❑	YES ❑ NO ❑			

*Does the triage level assigned meet the criteria as outlined by CTAS, ESI, MTS, ATS, or other designated triage acuity system?
**Auditing that the ECG was completed within 10 minutes of arrival is also important. This information may be indicated in the comments section but is often obtained utilizing a separate audit form.
ATS, Australasian Triage Scale; CTAS, Canadian Triage and Acuity Scale; ESI, Emergency Severity Index; MTS, Manchester Triage System.

Appendix E: Disaster Triage Tag

Appendix E: Disaster Triage Tag

☐ Personal Property
☐ Evidence Tag

00132001

Dest _____
Unit _____

00132001

REMOVE TO EXPOSE ADHESIVE

PEEL AND STICK TO PATIENT CHART

☐ Allergies ....

1-Abrasion
2-Amputation
3-Avulsion
4-Bleeding
5-Contusion
6-Puncture
7-Laceration
8-Pain
9-Deformity
10-Swelling
11-Other

Burn Reference

Head- 0%	Chest/Abd.
Arms- 9% each	Front -18%
Legs- 18% each	Rear- 18%

Place related minor or guardian labels here.

STATE OF NEW JERSEY

VICTIM DEMOGRAPHICS

Sex ☐ Information Unavailable
☐ M
☐ F Age_____ DOB_____ Wt_____ ☐ Lb. ☐ Kg.

Name ....
Address ....
City .... St ...... Zip ......
Phone ....
SSN ....
Religion ....

Triage *00132001*   Other *00132001*

Treat *00132001*   Other *00132001*

Trans *00132001*   Other *00132001*

DECEASED
00132001

IMMEDIATE
LIFE THREATENING INJURIES
00132001

DELAYED
NON-LIFE THREATENING INJURIES
00132001

MINOR
MINOR INJURIES
00132001

UNINJURED
DOCUMENTED BY OFFICIAL
00132001

Appendix E: Disaster Triage Tag

Personal Property / Evidence Tag — Attach stub or seal inside personal property or evidence bag

Patient Destination and Transport Unit — Remove this stub after arrival at hospital and keep until attached to patient care report

State of New Jersey Disaster Triage Tag

EMS-82 APR17 HS795

RESPIRATIONS R ☐ Yes ☐ No
PERFUSION P ☐ Pulse ☐ No
MENTAL STATUS M ☐ Can Do ☐ Can't Do

Condition	Triage
Move ANYONE ambulatory	MINOR
No Respiration after head tilt	DECEASED
Respirations OVER 30	IMMEDIATE
No radial pulse or Capillary refill over 2 Seconds	IMMEDIATE
Unable to follow simple commands	IMMEDIATE
Everyone else	DELAYED

☐ S Salivation ☐ L Lacrimation ☐ U Urination ☐ D Defecation ☐ G GI Distress ☐ E Emesis ☐ M Miosis

NAAK AUTO INJECTOR ☐ 1 ☐ 2 ☐ 3 ☐ 4 ☐ 5

☐ Dry Decon
☐ Gross Decon
☐ Technical Decon
Decon Solution _____
Circle Nature of Contaminant (Biological / Radiological / Chemical)

Chief Complaint:

Vitals

Time	B/P	Pulse	Resp	O₂ Sat.

Medications

Time	Medication	Dose	Route

IV Location _____ Ga. _____ Solution: _____ Rate: _____

Airway Adjunct _____ Size: _____ Depth: _____

STATE OF NEW JERSEY

DECEASED

IMMEDIATE
LIFE THREATENING INJURIES

DELAYED
NON-LIFE THREATENING INJURIES

MINOR
MINOR INJURIES

UNINJURED
DOCUMENTED BY OFFICIAL

Source: New Jersey Department of Health. (n.d.). State of New Jersey disaster triage tag. Retrieved from https://www.nj.gov/health/ems/triagetag.shtml

Additional Reading

Agency for Healthcare Research and Quality. (2014). *Team triage reduces emergency department walkouts, improves patient care.* Retrieved from https://innovations.ahrq.gov/profiles/team-triage-reduces-emergency-department-walkouts-improves-patient-care

American Association for the Surgery of Trauma. (n.d.). *Trauma facts.* Retrieved from http://www.aast.org/trauma-facts

American College of Cardiology/American Heart Association. (n.d.). *Guidelines and clinical documents.* Retrieved from http://www.acc.org/guidelines

American College of Emergency Physicians. (2018). *Clinical practice management guidelines.* Retrieved from https://www.acep.org/how-we-serve/sections/critical-care-medicine/resources/practice-guidelines/#sm.01pbnegm119lew011c12dwj9kmmj7

American College of Obstetricians and Gynecologists' Committee on Obstetric Practice; Macones, G. A., Pettker, C. M., Mascola, M. A., & Heine, R. P. (2016, July). *Committee opinion number 667: Hospital-based triage of obstetric patients.* Retrieved from http://www.acog.org/Resources-And-Publications/Committee-Opinions/Committee-on-Obstetric-Practice/Hospital-Based-Triage-of-Obstetric-Patients

American College of Surgeons. (2013, June 1). *Improving survival from active shooter events: The Hartford Consensus.* Retrieved from http://bulletin.facs.org/2013/06/improving-survival-from-active-shooter-events/#.Wz45KC2ZOMI

American Heart Association. (2018). *Stroke.* Retrieved from http://www.strokeassociation.org/STROKEORG/#

American Nurses Association. (2015). *Nursing: Scope and standards of practice* (3rd ed.). Silver Spring, MD: Author.

Amsterdam, E. A., Wenger, N. K., Brindis, R. G., Casey, D. E. Jr., Ganiats, T. G., Holmes, D. R. Jr., . . . Zieman, S. J. (2014). 2014 AHA/ACC guideline for the management of patients with non-ST-elevation acute coronary syndromes: Executive summary: A report of the American College of Cardiology/American Heart Association Task Force on Practice Guidelines. *Circulation, 130*(25), 2354–2394. doi:10.1161/CIR.0000000000000133

Anthony, B., Penrose, J. K., & Jakiel, S. (2017). *The typology of modern slavery: Defining sex and labor trafficking in the United States.* Washington, DC: Polaris. Retrieved at https://polarisproject.org/sites/default/files/Polaris-Typology-of-Modern-Slavery.pdf

Aston, J., Bull, N., Gschwandtner, U., Pflueger, M., Borgwardt, S., Stieglitz, R., & Riecher-Rössler, A. (2012). First self-perceived signs and symptoms in emerging psychosis compared with depression. *Early Intervention in Psychiatry, 6*(4), 455–459. doi:10.1111/j.1751-7893.2012.00354.x

Austin, S. (2006). "Ladies & gentlemen of the jury, I present…the nursing documentation." *Nursing, 36*(1), 56–62. doi:10.1097/00152193-200601000-00043

Australian Government Department of Health. (2009). *Emergency triage education kit.* Retrieved from http://www.health.gov.au

Baker, S. (2009). *Excellence in the emergency department: How to get results.* Gulf Breeze, FL: Firestarter.

Balentine, J. R., & Davis, C. P. (2013). *Human bites.* Retrieved from https://www.emedicinehealth.com/search/emh/human%20bites

Barbee, G., Berry-Caban, C., Daymude, M., Oliver, J., & Gay, S. (2012). The effect of provider level triage in a military treatment facility emergency department. *Australasian Journal of Paramedicine, 8*(4). Retrieved from https://ajp.paramedics.org/index.php/ajp/article/view/87/81

Becher, J., & Visovsky, C. (2012). Horizontal violence in nursing. *MedSurg Nursing, 21*(4), 210. Retrieved from https://www.amsn.org/sites/default/files/documents/practice-resources/healthy-work-environment/resources/MSNJ-Becher-Visovsky-21-04.pdf

Bemis, P. A. (2011). *Emergency nursing bible* (5th ed.). Huntington Beach, CA: National Nurses in Business Association.

Beveridge, R., Clarke, B., Janes, L., Savage, N., Thompson, J., Dodd, G., . . . Vadeboncoeur, A. (2018). *Implementation guidelines for the Canadian emergency department triage and acuity scale.* Retrieved from https://caep.ca/resources/ctas/implementation-guidelines

Billings, D. M., & Halstead, J. A. (2009). *Teaching in nursing: A guide for faculty* (3rd ed.). St. Louis, MO: Elsevier Saunders.

Blair, P. L. (2013). Lateral violence in nursing. *Journal of Emergency Nursing, 39*(5), e75. doi:10.1016/j.jen.2011.12.006

Blumberg, P. (2009). *Developing learner-centered teaching: A practical guide for faculty.* San Francisco, CA: Jossey-Bass.

Board of Certification for Emergency Nursing (BCEN). (2018). *Why certify?* Retrieved from https://www.bcencertifications.org/Get-Certified/Why-Certify

Boxer, B. A., & Boxer Goldfarb, E. M. (2009). The expectations and perceptions of ED patients. *Journal of Emergency Nursing, 35,* 540–541. doi:10.1016/j.jen.2007.08.025

Briggs, J. K. (2011). *Telephone triage protocols for nurses* (4th ed.). Philadelphia, PA: Lippincott.

Briggs, J. K., & Grossman, V. (2006). *Emergency nursing: 5-tier triage protocols*. Philadelphia, PA: Lippincott Williams & Wilkins.

Buettner, J. (2017). *Fast facts for the ER nurse: Emergency room orientation in a nutshell* (3rd ed.). New York, NY: Springer Publishing.

Bullard, M., Unger, B., Spence, J., Grafstein, E., & The CTAS National Working Group. (2008). Revisions to the Canadian emergency department triage and acuity. *Canadian Journal of Emergency Medicine, 10*(2), 136–142. doi:10.2310/8000.2014.012014

Campbell, J. (2012). *International trauma life support* (6th ed.). Boston, MA: Pearson.

Canadian Association of Emergency Physicians. (2018). *Canadian triage and acuity scale*. Retrieved from http://caep.ca/resources/ctas#support

Carper, K., & Machlin, S. R. (2018). *National health care expenses in the U.S. civilian noninstitutionalized population, 2010. Statistical brief #396*. Rockville, MD. Retrieved from https://meps.ahrq.gov/data_files/publications/st396/stat396.shtml

Castner, J., Grinslade, S., Guay, J., Hettinger, A. Z., Seo, J. Y., & Boris, L. (2013). Registered nurse scope of practice and ED complaint-specific protocols. *Journal of Emergency Nursing, 39*, 467–473. doi:10.1016/j.jen.2013.02.009

Center for Emergency Medicine Board Review. (2014). *19th annual the national emergency medicine board review course*. Retrieved from http://www.ccme.org/nembr

Centers for Disease Control and Prevention. (n.d.). *Guidance for the selection and use of personal protective equipment (PPE) in healthcare settings*. Retrieved from https://www.cdc.gov/HAI/pdfs/ppe/PPEslides6-29-04.pdf

Centers for Disease Control and Prevention. (2011). *National hospital ambulatory medical care survey: 2010 emergency department summary tables*. Retrieved from http://www.cdc.gov/nchs/data/ahcd/nhamcs_emergency/2010_ed_web_tables.pdf

Centers for Disease Control and Prevention. (2013). *Parasites—lice*. Retrieved from https://www.cdc.gov/parasites/lice/head/index.html

Centers for Disease Control and Prevention. (2017). *Smallpox basics*. Retrieved from https://www.cdc.gov/smallpox/index.html

Centers for Disease Control and Prevention. (2018a). *Ebola*. Retrieved from https://www.cdc.gov/vhf/ebola/outbreaks/drc/2018-may.html

Centers for Disease Control and Prevention. (2018b). *Immunization schedules*. Retrieved from https://www.cdc.gov/vaccines/schedules/index.html

Centers for Disease Control and Prevention. (2018c). *Transmission of measles*. Retrieved from https://www.cdc.gov/measles/about/transmission.html

Centers for Medicare & Medicaid Services. (2018a). *Promoting interoperability programs*. Retrieved from https://www.cms.gov/Regulations-and-Guidance/Legislation/EHRIncentivePrograms/index.html?redirect=/EHRIncentivePrograms

Ciocco, M. (2013). *Fast facts for the medical–surgical nurse: Clinical orientation in a nutshell*. New York, NY: Springer Publishing.

Colobong, J. V., & Watson, A. S. (2014). Caring for the patient with acute brain or cranial nerve disorder. In K. S. Osborn, C. E. Wraa, A. S. Watson, & R. S. Holleran (Eds.), *Medical surgical nursing: Preparation for practice* (2nd ed., pp. 503–551). Englewood Cliffs, NJ: Pearson/Prentice Hall.

Committee for Tactical Emergency Casualty Care. (2018). *Tactical emergency casualty care guidelines | C-TECC*. Retrieved from http://www.c-tecc.org

Considine, J., Lucas, E., Martin, R., Stergiou, H. E., Kropman, M., & Chiu, H. (2012). Rapid intervention and treatment zone: Redesigning nursing services to meet increasing emergency department demand. *International Journal of Nursing Practice, 18*, 60–67. doi:10.1111/j.1440-172X.2011.01986.x

Convoy, S., & Westphal, R. J. (2013). The importance of developing military cultural competence. *Journal of Emergency Nursing, 39*(6), 591–594. doi:10.1016/j.jen.2013.08.010

Cox, S., Smith, K., Currell, A., Harriss, L., Barger, B., & Cameron, P. (2011). Differentiation of confirmed major trauma patients and potential major trauma patients using pre-hospital triage criteria. *Injury, 42*, 889–895. doi:10.1016/j.injury.2010.03.035

Cushing, T. A., & Alcock, J. (2018). *Electrical injuries in emergency medicine clinical presentation*. Retrieved from https://emedicine.medscape.com/article/770179-clinical

Daniels, R. (2011). Surviving the first hours in sepsis: Getting the basics right (an intensivist's perspective). *Antimicrobial Chemotherapy, 66*(2), ii11–ii23. doi:10.1093/jac/dkq515

Dateo, J. (2013). What factors increase the accuracy and inter-rater reliability of the emergency severity index among emergency nurses in triaging adult patients? *Journal of Emergency Nursing, 39*(2), 203–207. doi:10.1016/j.jen.2011.09.002

Day, T., Al-Roubaie, A., & Goldlust, E. (2013). Decreased length of stay after addition of healthcare provider in emergency department triage. *Emergency Medicine Journal, 30*(2), 134–138. doi:10.1136/emermed-2012-201113

DeLemos, C., & Watson, A. S. (2014). Caring for the patient with cerebral vascular disorders. In K. S. Osborn, C. E. Wraa, A. S. Watson, & R. S. Holleran (Eds.), *Medical surgical nursing: Preparation for practice* (2nd ed., pp. 552–588). Englewood Cliffs, NJ: Pearson/Prentice Hall.

Dellinger, R., Levy, M., Rhodes, A., Djillali, A., Gerlach, H., Opal, S., . . . Surviving Sepsis Campaign Guidelines Committee Including the Pediatric Subgroup. (2013). Surviving sepsis campaign: International guidelines for management of severe sepsis and septic shock. *Critical Care Medicine, 41*, 580–637. doi:10.1097/CCM.0b013e31827e83af

Doerr, S., & Shiel, W. C. Jr. (2018). *Heat-related illness*. Retrieved from http://www.medicinenet.com/hyperthermia/article.htm

Drendel, A., Brousseau, D., & Gorelick, M. (2006). Pain assessment for pediatric patients in the emergency department. *Pediatrics, 117*(5), 1511–1518. doi:10.1542/peds.2005-2046

Ducharme, J. (2005). The future of pain management in emergency medicine. *Emergency Medicine Clinics of North America, 23*, 467–475. doi:10.1016/j.emc.2004.12.011

Edwards, T. (2013). *The art of triage.* Hauppauge, NY: Nova Science Publishers.

Emergency Nurses Association. (2001). *Making the right decision: A triage curriculum* (2nd ed.). Des Plaines, IL: Author.

Emergency Nurses Association. (2004). *Course in advanced trauma nursing II: A conceptual approach.* Des Plaines, IL: Author.

Emergency Nurses Association. (2007). *Emergency nursing core curriculum* (6th ed.). St. Louis, MO: Saunders.

Emergency Nurses Association. (2012). *Emergency nursing pediatric course: Provider manual* (4th ed.). Des Plaines, IL: Author.

Emergency Nurses Association. (2014a). *Disaster and emergency preparedness for all hazards* [Position statement]. Retrieved from https://www.ena.org/docs/default-source/resource-library/practice-resources/position-statements/allhazardspreparedness.pdf?sfvrsn=ea0879a4_10

Emergency Nurses Association. (2014b). *Emergency nursing certification.* Retrieved from https://www.ena.org/docs/default-source/resource-library/practice-resources/position-statements/encertification.pdf?sfvrsn=b3563eb6_12

Emergency Nurses Association. (2014c). *Patient experience/satisfaction in the emergency care setting.* Retrieved from https://www.ena.org/docs/default-source/resource-library/practice-resources/position-statements/patientexperiencesatisfactionined.pdf?sfvrsn=fa8cece1_8

Emergency Nurses Association. (2014d). *Trauma nursing core course provider manual* (7th ed.). Des Plaines, IL: Author.

Emergency Nurses Association. (2015a). *Emergency nurse orientation position statement.* Retrieved from https://www.ena.org/docs/default-source/resource-library/practice-resources/position-statements/emergencynurseorientation.pdf?sfvrsn=e3ee2b66_14

Emergency Nurses Association. (2015b). *Protection of human subjects position statement.* Retrieved from https://www.ena.org/docs/default-source/resource-library/practice-resources/position-statements/protectionofhumansubjects.pdf?sfvrsn=dbf151df_6

Emergency Nurses Association. (2015c). *Use of protocols in the emergency setting.* Retrieved from https://www.ena.org/docs/default-source/resource-library/practice-resources/position-statements/useofprotocolsined.pdf?sfvrsn=43f282ab_6

Emergency Nurses Association. (2016). *Weighing all patients in kilograms position statement.* Retrieved from https://www.ena.org/docs/default-source/resource-library/practice-resources/position-statements/weighingallpatientsinkilograms.pdf?sfvrsn=9c0709e_8

Emergency Nurses Association. (2017a). *Clinical practice guidelines: Synopsis suicide risk assessment*. Retrieved from https://www.ena.org/docs/default-source/resource-library/practice-resources/cpg/cpgsuicidesynopsis.pdf?sfvrsn=522e6ed5_18

Emergency Nurses Association. (2017b). *Emergency nursing triage course*. Retrieved from https://www.ena.org/education/onlinelearning/Pages/ENT.aspx

Emergency Nurses Association. (2017c). *Obstetrical patients in the emergency care setting position statement*. Retrieved from https://www.ena.org/docs/default-source/resource-library/practice-resources/position-statements/obpatientined.pdf?sfvrsn=e02a3d6c_12

Emergency Nurses Association. (2017d). *Triage qualifications and competency position statement*. Retrieved from https://www.ena.org/docs/default-source/resource-library/practice-resources/position-statements/triagequalificationscompetency.pdf?sfvrsn=a0bbc268_8

Emergency Nurses Association. (2018a). *Education*. Retrieved from https://www.ena.org/education

Emergency Nurses Association. (2018b). *ENA position statements*. Retrieved from https://www.ena.org/practice-resources/resource-library/position-statements

Emergency Nurses Association. (2018c). *Forensic evidence collection in the emergency care setting position statement*. Retrieved from https://www.ena.org/docs/default-source/resource-library/practice-resources/position-statements/forensic-evidence-collection-in-the-emergency-care-setting.pdf?sfvrsn=a1f89eba_4

Emergency Nurses Association and American College of Emergency Physicians. (2010). *Standardized ED triage scale and acuity categorization: Joint ENA/ACEP statement*. Retrieved from https://www.ena.org/SiteCollectionDocuments/Position%20Statements/Joint/StandardizedEDTriageScaleandAcuityCategorization.pdf

Evans, H., Summers, R., & Thompson, J. (2011). Implementing scripting in the emergency department: Does it measure up? *Annals of Emergency Medicine, 58*(4), S317. doi:10.1016/j.annemergmed.2011.06.442

Farrohknia, N., Castren, M., Ehrenberg, A., Lars, L., Oredsson, S., Jonsson, H., . . . Göransson, K. (2011). Emergency department triage scales and their components: A systematic review of the scientific evidence. *Scandinavian Journal of Trauma, Resuscitation & Emergency Medicine, 19*, 42. doi:10.1186/1757-7241-19-42

FitzGerald, G., Jelinek, G. A., Scott, D., & Gerdtz, M. F. (2010). Emergency department triage revisited. *Emergency Medicine Journal, 27*, 86–92. doi:10.1136/emj.2009.077081

Flanagan, M. (2005). Every patient deserves a safe nurse. *American Journal of Nursing, 105*(11), 112. doi:10.1097/00000446-200511000-00040

Foley, A. (2011). Talking the talk in triage. *Journal of Emergency Nursing, 37*(2), 205–206. doi:10.1016/j.jen.2010.11.009

Foley, A., & Durant, J. (2011). Let's ask that out front: Health and safety screening in triage. *Journal of Emergency Nursing, 37*(5), 515. doi:10.1016/j.jen.2011.06.013

Fosnocht, D. E., Swanson, E. R., & Barton, E. D. (2005). Changing attitudes about pain and pain control in emergency medicine. *Emergency Medicine Clinics of North America, 23,* 297–306. doi:10.1016/j.emc.2004.12.003

Foster, C. S. (2017). Stevens-Johnson syndrome treatment and management. In A. A. Dahl (Ed.), *Medscape.* Retrieved from http://emedicine.medscape.com/article/1197450-treatment

Gerdtz, M., & Bucknall, T. (1999). Why we do the things we do: Applying clinical decision-making frameworks to triage practice. *Accident and Emergency Nursing, 7*(1), 50–57. doi:10.1016/S0965-2302(99)80103-9

Gilboy, N., Tanabe, T., Travers, D., & Rosenau, A. M. (2011). *Emergency severity index (ESI): A triage tool for emergency department care, version 4. Implementation handbook 2012 edition* (AHRQ Publication No. 12-0014). Rockville, MD: Agency for Healthcare Research and Quality. Retrieved from http://www.ahrq.gov/sites/default/files/wysiwyg/professionals/systems/hospital/esi/esihandbk.pdf

Grossman, V. A. (2014). *Fast facts for the radiology nurse: An orientation and nursing care guide in a nutshell.* New York, NY: Springer Publishing.

Gutierrez, C., Lindor, R. A., Baker, O., Cutler, D., & Schuur, J. D. (2016). State regulation of freestanding emergency departments varies widely, affecting location, growth, and services provided. *Health Affairs, 35* (10), 1857–1866. doi:10.1377/hlthaff.2016.0412

Halliday, A. (2005). Creating a reliable time line. *Nursing, 35*(2), 27. doi:10.1097/00152193-200502000-00019

Hammond, B. B. (2012). Cardiovascular emergencies. In B. B. Hammond & P. G. Zimmermann (Eds.), *Sheehy's manual of emergency care* (7th ed.). St. Louis, MO: Elsevier.

Hammond, B. B., & Zimmermann, P. G. (Eds.). (2013). *Sheehy's manual of emergency care* (7th ed.). St. Louis, MO: Mosby.

Handel, D., Fu, R., Daya, M., York, J., Larson, E., & McConnell, K. (2010). The use of scripting at triage and its impact on elopements. *Academic Emergency Medicine, 17,* 495–500. doi:10.1111/j.1553-2712.2010.00721.x

Hayden, C., Burlingame, P., Thompson, H., & Sabol, V. (2013). Improving patient flow in the emergency department by placing a family nurse practitioner in triage: A quality improvement project. *Journal of Emergency Nursing, 40*(4), 346–351. doi:10.1016/j.jen.2013.09.011

Hohenhaus, S. (2006). Someone watching over me: Observations in pediatric triage. *Journal of Emergency Nursing, 32*(5), 398–403. doi:10.1016/j.jen.2006.07.002

Holleran, R. S., & Wraa, C. E. (2014). Caring for the patient with multisystem trauma. In K. S. Osborn, C. E. Wraa, A. S. Watson, & R. S. Holleran (Eds.), *Medical-surgical nursing: Preparation for practice* (2nd ed., pp. 2091–2112). Englewood Cliffs, NJ: Pearson/Prentice Hall.

Howard, P. K., & Steinmann, R. A. (Eds.). (2010). *Sheehy's emergency nursing: Principles and practice* (6th ed.). St. Louis, MO: Mosby.

Hoyt, K. S., & Selfridge-Thomas, J. (2007). *Emergency nursing core curriculum* (6th ed., pp. 459–460). Philadelphia, PA: Saunders/Elsevier.

Innes, K., Plummer, V., & Considine, V. (2011). Nurses' perceptions of their preparation for triage. *Australasian Emergency Nursing Journal, 14*(2), 81–86. doi:10.1016/j.aenj.2011.03.003

International Association for the Study of Pain. (1994). Part III: Pain terms, a current list with definitions and notes on usage. In H. Merskey and N. Bogduk (Eds.), *Classification of chronic pain, second edition, IASP task force on taxonomy* (pp. 209–214). Seattle, WA: IASP Press.

International Labour Organization. (2016). *Forced labour, modern slavery and human trafficking*. Retrieved from http://www.ilo.org/global/topics/forced-labour/lang--en/index.htm

Janiak, B. D. (2009, May 1). *Guest column: Tips to succeed in getting sued*. Retrieved from https://www.reliasmedia.com/articles/112833-guest-column-tips-to-succeed-in-getting-sued?utm_source=TrendMD&utm_medium=cpc&utm_campaign=AHC_Media_TrendMD_0

The Joint Commission. (2013). *Specifications manual for national hospital inpatient quality measures*. Retrieved from https://www.jointcommission.org/specifications_manual_for_national_hospital_inpatient_quality_measures.aspx

The Joint Commission Standards. (2018). *Standards information for hospitals*. Retrieved from https://www.jointcommission.org/accreditation/hap_standards_information.aspx

Jordi, K., Grossmann, F., Gaddis, G. M., Cignacco, E., Denhaerynck, K., Schwendimann, R., & Nickel, C. H. (2015). Nurses' accuracy and self-perceived ability using the Emergency Severity Index triage tool: A cross-sectional study in four Swiss hospitals. *Scandinavian Journal of Trauma, Resuscitation and Emergency Medicine, 23*, 62. doi:10.1186/s13049-015-0142-y

Kothari, R. U., Pancioli, A., Liu, T., Brott, T., & Broderick, J. (1999). Cincinnati Prehospital Stroke Scale: Reproducibility and validity. *Annals of Emergency Medicine, 33*(4), 373–378. doi:10.1016/S0196-0644(99)70299-4

Kroekel, P. A., George, L., & Eltoukhy, N. (2013). How to manage the patient in the emergency department with a left ventricular assist device. *Journal of Emergency Nursing, 39*(5), 447–453. doi:10.1016/j.jen.2012.01.007

Lavoie-Tremblay, M., Leclerc, E., Marchionni, C., & Drevniok, U. (2010). The needs and expectations of generation Y nurses in the workplace. *Journal for Nurses in Staff Development, 26*(1), 2–8. doi:10.1097/NND.0b013e3181a68951

Liedtke, B. (2013). The case for mentoring in emergency departments. *Australian College for Emergency Medicine*, version 1.1, 1–12.

Lombardo, B., & Eyre, C. (2011). Compassion fatigue: A nurse's primer. *Online Journal of Issues in Nursing, 16*(1), 3. doi:10.3912/OJIN.Vol16No01Man03

Lorenzi, N. M., Kouroubali, A., Detmer, D. E., & Bloomrosen, M. (2009). How to successfully select and implement electronic health records (EHR) in small ambulatory practice settings. *BMC Medical Informatics and Decision Making, 9,* 15–28. doi:10.1186/1472-6947-9-15

Love, R., Murphy, J., Lietz, T., & Jordan, K. (2012). The effectiveness of a provider in triage in the emergency department: A quality of improvement initiative to improve patient flow. *Advanced Emergency Nursing Journal, 34*(1), 65–74. doi:10.1097/TME.0b013e3182435543

Manchester Triage Group. (2014). *Emergency triage: Manchester triage group* (3rd ed.). Chichester: John Wiley.

Manchester Triage System. (n.d.). Retrieved from http://www.triagenet.net/en

MacWilliams, K., Hughes, J., Aston, M., Field, S., & Moffatt, F. W. (2016). Understanding the experience of miscarriage in the emergency department. *Journal of Emergency Nursing, 42*(6), 504–512. doi:10.1016/j.jen.2016.05.011

McCarthy, M., Zeger, S., Ding, R., Levin, S., Desmond, J., Lee, J., & Arnosky, D. (2009). Crowding delays treatment and lengthens emergency department length of stay, even among high-acuity patients. *Annals of Emergency Medicine, 54*(4), 492.e4–503.e4. doi:10.1016/j.annemergmed.2009.03.006

Morrison, K. J. (2014). *Fast facts for stroke care nursing: An expert guide in a nutshell.* New York, NY: Springer Publishing.

Muller, M. L. (2014). Pediatric bacterial meningitis. In R. W. Steele (Ed.), *Medscape.* Retrieved from https://emedicine.medscape.com/article/961497-overview

Murray, M., Bullard, M., & Grafstein, E.; CTAS National Working Group; CEDIS National Working Group. (2004). Revisions to the Canadian Emergency Department Triage and Acuity Scale implementation guidelines. *Canadian Journal of Emergency Medicine, 6*(6), 421–427. doi:10.1017/S1481803500009428

National Institute of Neurological Disorders and Stroke. (2011). *Guillain-Barre syndrome fact sheet.* NIH Pub. No. 11-2902. Retrieved from http://www.ninds.nih.gov/disorders/gbs/detail_gbs.htm

National Stroke Association. (n.d.). *Stroke resources.* Retrieved from http://www.stroke.org/stroke-resources?gclid=EAIaIQobChMIuPSrpYnX2wIVGNlkCh27MQ35EAAYASAAEgKm_vD_BwE

O'Gara, P. T., Kushner, F. G., Ascheim, D. D., Casey, D. E. Jr., Chung, M. K., de Lemos, J. A., . . . CF/AHA Task Force. (2013). 2013 ACCF/AHA guideline for the management of ST-elevation myocardial infarction: A report of the American College of Cardiology Foundation/American Heart Association Task Force on practice guidelines. *Circulation, 127*(4), 529–555. doi:10.1161/CIR.0b013e3182742c84

Pante, M., & Pollak, A. (Eds.) (2010). *Advanced assessment & treatment of trauma.* Boston, MA: Jones & Bartlett.

Pearson, H. (2013). Science and intuition: Do both have a place in clinical decision making? *British Journal of Nursing, 22*(4), 212–215. doi:10.12968/bjon.2013.22.4.212

Pich, J., Hazelton, M., Sundin, D., & Kable, A., (2011). Patient-related violence at triage: Qualitative descriptive study. *International Emergency Nursing, 19*, 12–19. doi:10.1016/j.ienj.2009.11.007

Pines, J. M., Hilton, J. A., Weber, E. J., Alkemade, A. J., Al Shabanah, H., Anderson, P. D., . . . Schull, M. J. (2011). International perspectives on emergency department crowding. *Academic Emergency Medicine, 18*, 1358–1370. doi:10.1111/j.1553-2712.2011.01235.x

Pines, J. M., & Hollander, J. (2008). Emergency department crowding is associated with poor care for patients with severe pain. *Annals of Emergency Medicine, 51*(1), 1–5. doi:10.1016/j.annemergmed.2007.07.008

Press Ganey. (2018). *Emergency department patient experience*. Retrieved from http://www.pressganey.com/resources/emergency-department-patient-experience

Randall, J. R., Colman, I., & Rowe, B. H. (2011). A systematic review of psychometric assessment of self-harm risk in the emergency department (structured abstract). *Journal of Affective Disorders, 134*(1), 348–355. doi:10.1016/j.jad.2011.05.032

Rehberg, S., Maybauer, M., Enkhbaatar, P., Maybauer, D., Yamamoto, Y., & Traber, D. (2010). Pathophysiology, management and treatment of smoke inhalation injury. *Expert Review of Respiratory Medicine, 3*(3), 282–297. doi:10.1586/ERS.09.21

Retezar, R., Bessman, E., Ding, R., Zeger, S. L., & McCarthy, M. L. (2011). The effect of triage diagnostic standing orders on emergency department treatment time. *Annals of Emergency Medicine, 57*(2), 89–99. doi:10.1016/j.annemergmed.2010.05.016

Robinson, D. J. (2013). An integrative review: Triage protocols and the effect on ED length of stay. *Journal of Emergency Nursing, 39*, 398–408. doi:10.1016/ j.jen.2011.12.016

Rowe, B. H., Villa-Roel, C., Guo, X., Bullard, M. J., Ospina, M., Vandermeer, B., . . . Holroyd, B. R. (2011). The role of triage nurse ordering on mitigating overcrowding in emergency departments: A systematic review. *Academic Emergency Medicine, 18*, 1349–1357. doi:10.1111/j.1553-2712.2011.01081.x

Russ, S., Jones, I., Aronsky, D., Dittus, R. S., & Slovis, C. M. (2010). Placing physician orders at triage: The effect on length of stay. *Annals of Emergency Medicine, 56*(1), 27–33. doi:10.1016/j.anneemergmed.2010.02.006

Rutenberg, C., & Greenberg, E. (2012). *The art and science of telephone triage: How to practice nursing over the phone*. Hot Springs, AR: Telephone Triage Consulting.

Ryan, K., Greenslade, J., Dalton, E., Chu, K., Brown, A. F. T., & Cullen, L. (2016). Factors associated with triage assignment of emergency department patients ultimately diagnosed with acute myocardial infarction. *Australian Critical Care, 29*(1), 23–26. doi:10.1016/j.aucc.2015.05.001

Sanchez, C., Valdez, A., & Johnson, L. (2014). Hoop dancing to prevent and decrease burnout and compassion fatigue. *Journal of Emergency Nursing, 40*(4), 394. doi:10.1016/j.jen.2014.04.013

Smith, E., Saver, J. L., Alexander, D. N., Furie, K. L., Hopkins, L. N., Katzan, I. L., . . . Williams, L. S. (2014). Clinical performance measures for adults hospitalized with acute ischemic stroke: Performance measures for healthcare professionals from the American Heart Association/American Stroke Association. *Stroke, 45*(11), 3472–3498. doi:10.1161/STR.0000000000000045

Stauber, M. A. (2013). Advanced nursing interventions and length of stay in the emergency department. *Journal of Emergency Nursing, 39*, 221–225. doi:10.1016/j.jen.2012.02.015

Studer, Q., Hagins, M., & Cochrane, B. (2014). The power of engagement: Creating the culture that gets your staff aligned and invested. *Healthcare Management Forum, 27*, S79–S87. doi:10.1016/j.hcmf.2014.01.008

Sulfaro, S. (2009). Charting the course for triage decisions. *Journal of Emergency Nursing, 35*(3), 268–269. doi:10.1016/jen.2009.01.003

Svinicki, M., & McKeachie, W. J. (2011). *McKeachie's teaching tips: Strategies, research, and theory for college and university teachers* (13th ed.). Belmont, CA: Wadsworth.

Thomas, D. O., & Bernardo, L. M. (Eds.). (2009). *Core curriculum for pediatric emergency nursing* (2nd ed.). Des Plaines, IL: Emergency Nurses Association.

Tintinalli, J. E., Kelen, G. D., & Stapczynski, J. S. (2004). *Emergency medicine: A comprehensive study guide* (6th ed.). New York, NY: McGraw-Hill.

Tipsord-Klinkhammer, B., & Andreoni, C. P. (1998). *Quick reference to emergency nursing*. Philadelphia, PA: W. B. Saunders.

Triage First, Inc. (2012). *ED triage comprehensive course; ED triage systematics, documentation lecture*. Asheville, NC: Author.

Triage First. (2018). *ED triage comprehensive course*. Retrieved from http://www.triagefirst.com/ed-triage-comprehensive-course

U.S. Department of Health and Human Services. (n.d.). *CDC blast injuries and patterns of care-fact sheet for professionals*. Retrieved from http://emergency.cdc.gov/masscasualties/pdf/blast_fact_sheet_professionals-a.pdf

U.S. Department of Health and Human Services. (2017). *START mass casualty triage algorithm*. Retrieved from https://chemm.nlm.nih.gov/StartAdultTriageAlgorithm.pdf

U.S. Department of Health and Human Services. (2017a). *A decision makers guide: Medical planning and response for a nuclear detonation*. Retrieved from https://www.remm.nlm.gov/decisionmakersguide.htm

U.S. Department of Health and Human Services. (2017b). *SALT mass casualty triage algorithm*. Retrieved from https://remm.nlm.nih.gov/salttriage.htm

U.S. Department of Health and Human Services. (2018a). *Primary response incident scene management (PRISM) decontamination guidance for chemical incidents*. Retrieved from https://www.medicalcountermeasures.gov/barda/cbrn/prism

U.S. Department of Health and Human Services. (2018b). *Topic collection: On-scene mass casualty triage and trauma care.* Retrieved from https://asprtracie.hhs.gov/technical-resources/33/on-scene-mass-casualty-triage-and-trauma-care/27

U.S. Department of Justice. (2017). *National strategy to combat human trafficking.* Retrieved from https://www.justice.gov/humantrafficking/page/file/922791/download

U.S. Department of Labor. (n.d.). *Hazardous waste operations and emergency response.* U.S. Code of Regulations 29 CFR 1910.120(q). Retrieved from https://www.osha.gov/pls/oshaweb/owadisp.show_document?p_table=STANDARDS&p_id=9765

U.S. Department of State. (2017). *2017 trafficking in persons report.* Retrieved from https://www.state.gov/j/tip/rls/tiprpt

Vartak, S., Crandall, D. K., Brokel, J. M., Wakefield, D. S., & Ward, M. M. (2009). Professional practice and innovation: Transformation of emergency department processes of care with EHR, CPOE, and ER even tracking. *Health Information Management Journal, 38*(2), 27–32. doi:10.1177/183335830903800204

Visser, L., & Montejano, A. (2018). *Rapid access guide for triage and emergency nurses: Chief complaints with high risk presentations.* New York, NY: Springer Publishing.

Vitulano, N., Riccioni, G., & Trivisano, A. (2012). Atypical presentation of acute coronary syndrome–not ST elevation: A case report. *Care Reports in Medicine, 2012*, 182379. doi:10.1155/2012/182379

Vuille, M., Foerrster, M., Foucalt, E., & Hugli, O. (2017). Pain assessment by emergency nurses at triage in the emergency department: A qualitative study. *Journal of Clinical Nursing, 27*, 669–676. doi:10.1111/jocn.13992

Warren, D. W., Jarvis, A., Le Blanc, L., Gravel, J., & CTAS National Working Group. (2008). Revisions to the Canadian triage & acuity scale paediatric guidelines (PaedCTAS). *Canadian Journal of Emergency Medicine, 10*(3), 224–232. doi:10.1017/S1481803500010149

Weingarten, R. M., & Weingarten, C. T. (2013). Generational diversity in ED and education settings: A daughter–mother perspective. *Journal of Emergency Nursing, 39*(4), 369–371. doi:10.1016/j.jen.2013.05.008

Welch, S. (2008). Preventing ED violence starts in triage. *Emergency Medicine News, 30*(12), 4. doi:10.1097/01.EEM.0000342733.39531.17

Wiler, J., Gentle, C., Halfpenny, J., Heins, A., Mehrotra, A., Mikhail, M., & Fite, D. (2009). Optimizing emergency department front-end operations. *Annals of Emergency Medicine, 55*(2), 142–160. doi:10.1016/j.annemergmed.2009.05.021

Wishner, J., & Burton, R. (2017). *How have providers responded to the increased demand for health care under the affordable care act?* Princeton, NJ: Robert Wood Johnson Foundation.

World Health Organization. (2005). *Emergency triage assessment and treatment (ETAT) course: Manual for participants.* Geneva, Switzerland: Author. Retrieved from http://www.who.int/maternal_child_adolescent/documents/9241546875/en

World Health Organization. (2016). *Paediatric emergency triage, assessment and treatment: Care of critically ill children.* Geneva, Switzerland: Author. Retrieved from http://www.who.int/maternal_child_adolescent/documents/paediatric-emergency-triage-update/en

Yang, C. Y., Liu, H. Y., Lin, H. L., & Lin, J. N. (2012). Left-sided acute appendicitis: A pitfall in the emergency department. *Journal of Emergency Medicine, 43*(6), 980–982. doi:10.1016/j.jemermed.2010.11.056

Zimmermann, P. G., & Herr, R. D. (2006). *Triage nursing secrets.* St. Louis, MO: Elsevier.

Index

abdominal aortic aneurysm, 148
abdominal aortic dissection, 136
abdominal emergencies, 145–151
    abdominal aortic aneurysm, 148
    appendicitis, 149
    cholecystitis, 149
    diverticulitis, 149
    esophageal varices, 149
    generic assessment
        abdominal assessment, 147–148
        skin assessment, 147
        vital signs, 147
    generic interventions, 148
    generic questions, 146–147
    GI bleeding, 150
    incarcerated hernia, 150
    large intestinal obstruction, 151
    pancreatitis, 151
    penile fracture, 151
    peptic ulcer disease, 151
    priapism, 152
    red flag findings, 145
    small intestinal obstruction, 151
    testicular torsion, 152
    worst-case scenarios, 146
abdominal pain, 114
abdominal trauma, 190–191
abruptio placentae, 155–156
abuse
    alcohol, 237
    child, 217
    elder, 225–226
    physical, 234
    substance, 237
    verbal, 233
access to information, 99
ACLS. *See* advanced cardiac life support
across-the-room assessment, 42–43, 120
active shooter/active violence, 255–262
    bleeding, stopping, 261–262
    critical incident stress management, 262
    incident response, 258–260
        community, attack occurring within, 258
        department/unit, attack occurring outside, 260
        department/unit, attack occurring within, 259–260
        hospital/healthcare facility, attack occurring within, 259
        preparation for law enforcement response, 260
    incident statistics of, 257
    preparation, 255–256

active shooter/active violence (*cont.*)
 situational awareness, 256–258
  behavioral warning signs, 256–257
  informational leakage warning signs and statistics, 257
  weapon concealment, 258
acute angle-closure glaucoma, 169
acute coronary syndrome (ACS), 134–136
acute myocardial infarction (AMI), 82–84
 nursing actions at triage, 83–84
 risk factors for, 82
 screening questions/assessment, 82
 treatment goals for, 82–83
acute pain, 230
ADLS. *See* advanced disaster life support
adolescent (13–18 years), development, 213
adrenal crisis, 178
adult teaching and learning principles, 11–13
 learning styles, 12
 orientee, supporting, 13
 right questions, asking, 12–13
advanced cardiac life support (ACLS), 5
advanced disaster life support (ADLS), 5
advanced triage protocols (ATPs), 111–116
 abdominal pain, 114
 altered level of consciousness, 114–115
 chest pain, 115–116
 considerations and concerns, 112–114
 defined, 111
 educational requirements for initiating, 113–114
 extremity injury, 115
 fever, 115
 initiation of, 112–113
 key aspects of, 112
 neurological symptoms, 115–116
 pain management, 116
 psychological complaints, 116
 reasons for using, 112
 reviewing results, 113
 shortness of breath, 116
 vaginal bleeding, 116
against medical advice (AMA), 62, 78
agitation
 emergency department staff, role of, 236
 situational reasons for, 234–236
airway, breathing, circulation, disability, and exposure (ABCDE), 216
alcohol abuse, 237
altered level of consciousness (ALOC), 114–115
American College of Cardiology, 84
American Heart Association, 84
 Guidelines for the Early Management of Patients with Acute Ischemic Stroke (2018), 85
AMI. *See* acute myocardial infarction
amniotic fluid leaking/ruptured membrane, 156
amputation, 175
anaphylaxis, 127
aortic dissection, 136
appendicitis, 149
arrhythmia, 134
arterial bleeding, 175
arterial occlusion, 175
Australasian Triage Scale (ATS), 35, 69, 72–73
AVPU (alert, verbal, pain, unresponsive), 123

baby boomers, 13, 14
basic disaster life support (BDLS), 5
basic life support (BLS), 5
behavioral health emergencies, 161–165

danger to others, 163
generic assessment, 162
generic interventions, 162
generic questions, 162
manic behavior, 163
overdose, 164
psychotic episode, 164
red flag findings, 161–162
suicide, 164–165
worst-case scenarios, 162
behavioral health patients, 237
behavioral warning signs, 256–257
bites, 183
bleeding
arterial, 175
GI, 150
stopping, 261–262
vaginal, 116
BLS. *See* basic life support
blunt injuries, 189
bronchiolitis, 217
burns, 192

Canadian Triage and Acuity Scale (CTAS), 35, 69, 70, 72
cardiac emergencies, 134–137
acute coronary syndrome, 135–136
aortic dissection, 136
endocarditis, 137
generic assessment, 135
generic interventions, 135
generic questions, 134
pericardial tamponade, 137
pericarditis, 137
worst-case scenarios, 134
case studies
diarrhea, 242
feeling funny, 243–244
foot pain, 244
inmate, 242–243
newborn not eating, 241–242
suicidal patient, 243
CAT. *See* combat application tourniquet
"caught ya" cards, 51
CEN. *See* certified emergency nurse

Centers for Medicare and Medicaid Services, 84
central retinal artery occlusion, 169
certifications, 5
certified emergency nurse (CEN), 5, 22, 24
certified pediatric emergency nurse (CPEN), 5
charge nurse and triage nurse, communication between, 104
chart audits
by others, 37
for self-review, 36–37
chemical burns to eye, 170
chest pain, 115–116
chickenpox, 196
chief complaint
electronic medical record, 98
eliciting, 120
subjective assessment of, 76
symptom-driven, 76
child abuse, 217
cholecystitis, 149
chronic pain, 230
C-I-AM-PEDS ("see, I am a kid"), 214
Cincinnati Prehospital Stroke Scale, 86
COBRA. *See* Consolidated Omnibus Budget Reconciliation Act of 1985
combat application tourniquet (CAT), 261–262
communication, 8–9, 54, 103–105
electronic medical record, 98
miscommunication, 234
with older adult patient, 223–224
between triage nurse and charge nurse/patient flow coordinator, 104
between triage staff and other departments, 104
between triage staff and patients/support systems, 104–105
within triage team, 103
compartment syndrome, 175

compassion fatigue, 29–30
  populations vulnerable to, 30
  prevention of, 30
  signs and symptoms of, 30
competency
  defined, 34
  education vs., 33–34
comprehensive triage assessment, 45–47
  information obtained during, 46
  longer assessment, reasons for, 46
consent to treatment, 61–62
Consolidated Omnibus Budget Reconciliation Act of 1985 (COBRA), 59–60
core measures, time-sensitive medical conditions, 81–82
CPEN. *See* certified pediatric emergency nurse
critical incident stress management, 262
critical thinking skills, 47–48
  examples of, 48
croup, 217
CTAS. *See* Canadian Triage and Acuity Scale
cultural competence, 226
current knowledge, advancing, 6
customer experience, in triage nursing, 49–57
  care for staff, 50
  communication, 54
  positive staff recognition, 50–51
  reassessments, 55–56
  rounding, 55
  scripting, 52–54
  service excellence, training for, 51–52
  service excellence efforts, evaluation of, 57
  service recovery, 56–57

decontamination control zones, 251
delay in care, 43
detached retina, 170
developmentally delayed patients, 209

diabetic ketoacidosis, 179
diarrhea, 242
disaster drills and exercises, 249
diverticulitis, 145
documentation, 76–80
  essential components of, 76–78
    arrival time, 76
    assessment statement, 77
    evaluation, 77
    interventions, 77
    objective triage assessment, 77
    plan, 77
    reassessments, 78
    subjective assessment of chief complaint, 76
    time seen by triage nurse, 76
  left prior to medical screening exam (LPMSE), 78
  left without being seen (LWBS), 78
  left without treatment (LWT), 78
  against medical advice (AMA), 78
  mnemonics, 78–79
  skills, enhancing, 6
drug overdose, risk for, 231
dysrhythmia. *See* arrhythmia

Ebola virus disease, 194–195
eclampsia, 157
ectopic pregnancy, 156
ED. *See* emergency management
education
  vs. competency, 33–34
  defined, 34
elder abuse, 225–226
electrocution, 184
electronic medical record (EMR), 7, 9, 15, 16, 97–100
  benefits of, 97–99
    access to information, 99
    chief complaint, 98
    communication, 98
  pitfalls of, 100
    downtime and upgrades, 100
    layout, 100
EMC. *See* emergency medical condition

emergency management (ED), 247–254
  phases of, 248
    mitigation, 248
    preparedness, 248–249
    recovery, 253–254
    response, 249–252
emergency medical condition (EMC), 60
Emergency Medical Treatment and Active Labor Act (EMTALA), 7, 16, 52, 59–61, 63, 94
  medical screening exam (MSE), 60
  pitfalls of, 61
emergency nurse pediatric course (ENPC), 5
Emergency Nurses Association (ENA), 4, 5, 33
emergency operations plan (EOP), 248–249
Emergency Severity Index (ESI), 35, 69, 70, 72
empathy burnout, 32
  impact on patient safety, 32
  prevention of, 32
EMR. *See* electronic medical record
encephalitis, 141
endocarditis, 137
endocrine emergencies, 177–180
  adrenal crisis, 178
  diabetic ketoacidosis, 179
  generic assessment, 178
  generic interventions, 178
  generic questions, 178
  hyperosmolar hyperglycemic state (HHS), 179
  hypoglycemia, 179
  thyroid storm, 180
  worst-case scenarios, 177
environmental emergencies, 181–185
  bites, 183
  electrocution, 184
  generic assessment, 182
  generic interventions, 182–183
  generic questions, 182
  hyperthermia, 184
  hypothermia, 184
  red flag findings, 181–182
  snake bite, 183
  stings, 184
  submersion, 185
  worst-case scenarios, 182
EOP. *See* emergency operations plan
epidermal necrolysis, 196
epiglottitis, 127–128
equipment lists, 9
ESI. *See* Emergency Severity Index
esophageal varices, 149–150
expressed consent, 61
extremity injury, 115
extremity trauma, 191
eye. *See also* ocular emergencies
  blunt trauma to, 169
  chemical burns to, 170
  trauma, penetrating, 171

feeling funny, 243–244
fever, 115
flesh-eating disease, 197–198
foot pain, 244
foreign body/abrasion, eye, 170
foreign body aspiration/obstruction, 218
  partial or complete, 128

GENE. *See* geriatric emergency nurse education
generation X, 13, 14
generation Y, 13, 14
generational divide, 13–15
geriatric emergency nurse education (GENE), 5
GI bleeding, 150
Glasgow Coma Scale (GCS), 43, 99, 123
Guidelines for the Early Management of Patients with Acute Ischemic Stroke (2018), 85
Guillain–Barré syndrome, 142
gynecological emergencies. *See* obstetric and gynecological emergencies

hazard vulnerability assessment (HVA), 248
hazardous materials (hazmat), 250
head trauma, 191
Health Insurance Portability and Accountability Act of 1996 (HIPAA), 7, 63, 64
  privacy requirements, meeting, 63–64
hearing-impaired patient, 207
HELLP syndrome, 157
hernia, incarcerated, 150
HHS. *See* hyperosmolar hyperglycemic state
high-pressure injury, 176
horizontal violence. *See* lateral violence
hospital incident command system (HICS), 249
hospital recovery, 254
human trafficking, 201–203
  exhibit, what victims may, 202
  tips to nurse, for reorganizing victims, 202–203
  victim, suggestions for recognizing, 202
hyperosmolar hyperglycemic state (HHS), 179
hyperthermia, 184
hypoglycemia, 179
hypothermia, 184

illiterate patient, 208
immediate bedding, 44–45
  criteria for practicing, 44
imminent delivery, 156–157
impetigo, 196
implied consent, 61
incarcerated hernia, 150
incident response, 258
  community, attack occurring in, 258
  department/unit, attack occurring outside, 260
  department/unit, attack occurring within, 259–260
  hospital/healthcare facility, attack occurring within, 259
  preparation for law enforcement response, 260
infant (birth–1 year), development, 212
infectious presentations, 193–198
  conditions requiring isolation, 196–198
  generic assessment, 195
  generic interventions, 195
  generic questions, 194
  red flag findings, 193–194
informational leakage warning signs and statistics, 257
informed consent, 62
inhalation injury, 128
injuries
  blunt, 189
  extremity, 115
  high-pressure, 176
  inhalation, 128
  orthopedic, 189
  penetrating, 189
inmate, 242–243
insulin, 179
insurance, 235
intestinal obstruction
  large, 151
  small, 151
intimate partner violence (IPV), 203–204
intussusceptions, 218
involuntary consent, 61

Joint Commission, 84

language barrier, patient with, 208–209
large intestinal obstruction, 151
lateral violence, 31–32
  consequences of, 31
  forms of, 31
  prevention of, 31–32
law enforcement response, preparation for, 260

learning styles, 12
left before treatment complete (LBTC), 62
left prior to the MSE (LPMSE), 62, 78
left ventricular assist devices (LVADs), patients with, 206–207
  complications in, 206
  normal findings in, 206
  suggestions to assist, 206–207
left without being seen (LWBS), 62, 78
left without treatment (LWT), 62, 78
legal concerns, in triage nursing, 59–64, 63–64
  consent to treatment, 61–62
  Emergency Medical Treatment and Active Labor Act (EMTALA), 59–61
  reportable conditions and events, 64
lesbian, gay, bisexual, transgender, questioning/queer (LGBTQ), 205–206
lice, 196
life-threatening bleeding, identifying, 261
Los Angeles Prehospital Stroke Screen, 86
Ludwig's angina, 128

management of aggressive behavior (MOAB), 236
Manchester Triage System (MTS), 69, 73
manic behavior, 163
multi-casualty incident (MCI)
  hazardous material incidents, 250–251
  MCI/disaster triage, 252, 275–277
  medical incidents, 249–250
  trauma incidents, 249
measles, 196
medical screening exam (MSE), 7, 60

meningitis, 141, 197
military personnel, 204–205
miscommunication, 234
mistriage, 71
  avoiding, 71
  causes of, 71
mitigation, emergency management, 248
motor vehicle crash (MVC), 79
MSE. *See* medical screening exam
musculoskeletal emergencies, 173–176
  amputation, 175
  arterial bleeding, 175
  arterial occlusion, 175
  compartment syndrome, 175
  generic assessment, 174
  generic interventions, 174
  generic questions, 174
  high-pressure injury, 176
  neurovascular compromise, 176
  red flag findings, 173
  worst-case scenarios, 174
MVC. *See* motor vehicle crash

National Institutes of Health Stroke Scale (NIHSS), 86
negative customer experiences, 56–57
  resolving, 57
  service recovery for, 56–57
neurological emergencies, 139–143
  encephalitis, 141
  generic assessment, 140
  generic interventions, 141
  generic questions, 140
  Guillain-Barré syndrome, 142
  meningitis/encephalitis, 141
  red flag findings, 139–140
  seizures, 142
  stroke, 143
  worst-case scenarios, 140
neurological symptoms, 115–116
neurovascular compromise, 176
newborn not eating, 241–242
nursemaid's elbow, 218
nurse's intuition, examples of, 48

nursing educators, 18–19
nursing leadership, 18–19

objective triage assessment, of documentation, 77
obstetric and gynecological emergencies, 153–160
    abruptio placentae, 155–156
    amniotic fluid leaking/ruptured membrane, 156
    eclampsia, 157
    ectopic pregnancy, 156
    generic assessment, 155
    generic interventions, 155
    generic questions, 154–155
    HELLP syndrome, 157
    imminent delivery, 156–157
    ovarian torsion, 158–159
    placenta previa, 157
    preeclampsia, 157
    prolapsed cord, 158
    red flag findings, 154
    sexual assault, 159
    toxic shock syndrome, 160
    trauma in pregnancy greater than 24 weeks, 158
    uterine rupture, 158
    worst-case scenarios, 154
ocular emergencies, 167–171
    acute angle-closure glaucoma, 169
    blunt trauma, 169
    central retinal artery occlusion, 169
    chemical burns, 170
    detached retina, 170
    foreign body/abrasion, 170
    generic assessment, 168
    generic interventions, 168
    generic questions, 168
    orbital cellulitis, 170
    penetrating eye trauma, 171
    red flag findings, 167–168
    ruptured globe, 171
    worst-case scenarios, 168
OLD CART, 78–79
older adult trauma, 191
older adult triage, 221–226
    assessment, 222
        emotional changes, 222
        physical changes, 222
        potential risks, 222
    atypical presentation, 225
    communication with patient, 223–224
    cultural competence, 226
    elder abuse, 225–226
    examination tips, 224
    polypharmacy, 225
orbital cellulitis, 170
orientee
    crucial conversations, 17–18
    giving praise, 18
    supporting, 13
orientation, 7–10
    communication, 8–9
    completion of, 9–10, 17–18
    equipment lists, 9
    evaluation techniques, 17
    policies and procedures, 16
    purpose of
        current knowledge, advancing, 6
        documentation skills, enhancing, 6
        policies and procedures, understanding, 7
        "red flag" patient presentations, identifying, 7
        triage flow, understanding, 6
        triage role, understanding, 6
    resources for, 10, 16
    right preceptors for, selecting, 8
    skills and processes, 16–17
    teamwork, 9
orthopedic injuries, 189
ovarian torsion, 158–159
overdose, 164
overreacting of parents, 211

pain, defined, 229
pain management, 116, 229–231
    acute pain, 230

chronic pain, 230
pain assessment, 230–231
red flag findings, 231
PALS. *See* pediatric advanced life support
pancreatitis, 151
patient acuity level, 122
patient arrival, 41–48
   comprehensive triage assessment, 45–47
   critical thinking skills, 47–48
   immediate bedding, 44–45
   rapid triage assessment, 42–43
   triage nurse, roles of, 41–42
patient experience, in triage nursing, 49–57
   care for staff, 50
   communication, 54
   positive staff recognition, 50–51
   reassessments, 55–56
   rounding, 55
   scripting, 52–54
   service excellence, training for, 51–52
   service excellence efforts, evaluation of, 57
   service recovery, 56–57
patient flow coordinator and triage nurse, communication between, 104
patient interview, 120
pediatric advanced life support (PALS), 5
Pediatric Assessment Triangle (PAT), 214
pediatric trauma, 191
pediatric triage, 211–218
   C-I-AM-PEDS ("see, I am a kid"), 214
   developmental stages
      adolescent (13–18 years), 213
      infant (birth–1 year), 212
      preschooler (3–5 years), 212
      school age (6–12 years), 212
      toddler (1–3 years), 212
   initial assessment, 213–214
   overview of, 211–212
   presentations, perils of, 216–218
      apparent life-threatening event, 216–217
      bronchiolitis, 217
      child abuse, 217
      croup, 217
      fever, 217
      foreign body aspiration, 218
      foreign body obstruction, 218
      intussusceptions, 218
      nursemaid's elbow, 218
      pyloric stenosis, 218
   vital signs, 215
pelvic inflammatory disease (PID) shuffle, 147
penetrating injuries, 189
penile fracture, 151
peptic ulcer disease, 151
pericardial tamponade, 137
pericarditis, 137
peritonsillar abscess, 128–129
personal awareness, for triage nurse, 29–32
   compassion fatigue, 29–30
   empathy burnout, 32
   lateral violence, 31–32
personal health information (PHI), protecting, 63
pertussis (whooping cough), 129
physical abuse, 234
physical assessment, 120–121
physical violence, 31
placenta previa, 157
pneumonia, 86–87, 129
   nursing actions at triage, 87
   risk factors for, 87
   screening questions/assessment, 87
   treatment goals for, 87
policies and procedures, 16
   understanding, 7
polypharmacy, 225
positive staff recognition, 50–51
PQRST, 23, 78–79, 82, 123
praise, 18
precepting at triage, 11–19
   adult teaching and learning principles, 11–13

precepting at triage (*cont.*)
  benefits of, 15
  generational divide, 13–15
  nursing leadership and educators, tips for, 18–19
  orientation
    completion of, 17–18
    ideas for, 16–17
  triage preceptor, desired traits in, 15
preeclampsia, 157
pregnancy
  ectopic, 156
  greater than 24 weeks, trauma in, 158
preparedness, emergency management, 248–249
preschooler (3–5 years), development, 212
priapism, 152
prolapsed cord, 158
provider in triage, 101–109
  key tips for, 105–107
  program, implementation of, 108–109
  purpose of placing, 101–102
psychological complaints, 116
psychological violence, 31
psychotic episode, 164
pulmonary embolism, 129–130
pyloric stenosis, 218

qualified medical person (QMP), 60

rapid triage assessment, 42–43
  delay in care, 43
reassessments, 55–56
  documentation, 78
recovery, emergency management, 253–254
red flag patient presentations, 119–124
  findings, 122
    abdominal emergencies, 15
    behavioral health emergencies, 161–162
    environmental emergencies, 181–182
    infectious presentations, 193–194
    musculoskeletal emergencies, 173
    neurological emergencies, 139–140
    obstetric and gynecological emergencies, 154
    ocular emergencies, 167–168
    pain management at triage, 231
    respiratory emergencies, 125–126
    trauma emergencies, 187–188
  generic assessment, 123
  generic interventions, 123–124
  generic questions, 123
  identifying, 7
  specific conditions, 124
  triage process, 120–122
    across-the-room assessment, 120
    chief complaint, eliciting, 120
    patient acuity level, 122
    patient interview, 120
    physical assessment, 120–121
    vital signs, 121
    worst-case scenarios, 122
reflection, 27
reportable conditions and events, 64
respiratory distress/respiratory failure, 130
respiratory emergencies, 125–131
  anaphylaxis, 127
  epiglottitis, 127–128
  foreign body obstruction, partial or complete, 128
  generic assessment, 126
  generic interventions, 127
  generic questions, 126
  inhalation injury, 128
  Ludwig's angina, 128
  peritonsillar abscess, 128–129
  pertussis (whooping cough), 129
  pneumonia, 129

pulmonary embolism, 129–130
red flag findings, 125
respiratory distress/respiratory failure, 130
tension pneumothorax, 130
tuberculosis, 130
worst-case scenarios, 126
response, emergency management, 249–253
retail medical clinics (RMCs), 95, 96
retrospective chart review, 36–37
by others, 37
for self-review, 36–37
right preceptors for triage orientation, selecting, 8
right questions, asking, 12–13
rounding, 55
rubella, 197
rubeola, 196
ruptured globe, 171

safety in triage area, increasing, 238–239
scabies, 197
school age (6–12 years), development, 212
scripting, 52–54
directions, 53
drinks, 53
status improvement during waiting time, 53–54
wait times, 52–53
security, 237–238
seizures, 142
self-security check, 258
sepsis, 88–89
nursing actions at triage, 89–90
risk factors for, 89
screening questions/assessment, 88–89
treatment goals for, 89
septic shock, 88–89
nursing actions at triage, 89–90
risk factors for, 89
screening questions/assessment, 88–89
treatment goals for, 89

service excellence, training for, 51–52
service excellence efforts, evaluation of, 57
service recovery, 56–57
severe sepsis, 88–89
nursing actions at triage, 89–90
risk factors for, 89
screening questions/assessment, 88–89
treatment goals for, 89
sexual assault, 159
shingles, 197
shortness of breath, 116
situational awareness, 256–260
behavioral warning signs, 256–257
informational leakage warning signs and statistics, 257
weapon concealment, 258
small intestinal obstruction, 151
smallpox, 197
snake bite, 183
SOAP (Subjective, Objective, Assessment, Plan), 76
sort, assess, lifesaving interventions, triage and/or transport (SALT) triage, 252
spinal trauma, 191
staff/personal recovery, 254
staff(ing)
care for, 50
positive staff recognition, 50–51
role, at triage, 102–103
triage. *See* triage staff
urgent care centers (UCC), 94
Stevens–Johnson syndrome, 196
stings, 184
stop-the-bleed training, 261–262
stroke, 84–86, 143
nursing actions at triage, 86
risk factors for, 85
screening questions/assessment, 84
treatment goals for, 85–86
subjective assessment of chief complaint, 76
submersion, 185

substance abuse, 237
sufficient severity, 60
suicidal patient, 243
suicide, 164–165
Suicide Risk Assessment, 162
Surviving Sepsis Campaign, 90

teamwork, 9
tension pneumothorax, 130
testicular torsion, 152
thoracic aortic dissection, 136
thyroid storm, 180
time-sensitive medical conditions, 81–90
    acute myocardial infarction, 82–84
    core measures, 81–82
    other/up-and-coming, 88
    pneumonia, 86–87
    sepsis, 88–89
    septic shock, 88–89
    severe sepsis, 88–89
    stroke, 84–86
TNCC. *See* trauma nurse core course
toddler (1–3 years), development, 212
toxic shock syndrome, 160
toxidromes, 250
trauma
    blunt trauma to eyes, 169
    penetrating eye, 171
    in pregnancy greater than 24 weeks, 158
trauma emergencies, 187–192
    abdominal trauma, 190–191
    blunt injuries, 189
    burns, 192
    chest, 191
    extremity trauma, 191
    generic assessment, 189
        airway, 189
        breathing, 189
        circulation, 189
        disability, 189
        history, 189
        injuries, 189
    generic interventions, 190
    generic questions, 188
        mechanism of injury, 188
    head trauma, 191
    older adult trauma, 191
    orthopedic injuries, 189
    pediatric trauma, 191
    penetrating injuries, 189
    red flag findings, 187–188
    spinal trauma, 191
    victims of violence, 192
    worst-case scenarios, 188
trauma nurse core course (TNCC), 5
triage
    advanced protocols, 111–116
    area safety, increasing, 238
    comprehensive assessment, 45–47
    defined, 4
    pediatric, 211–218
    precepting at. *See* precepting at triage
    provider in, 101–109
    qualifications, 4–5
    rapid assessment, 42–43
    staff. *See* triage staff
    team, communication within, 103
    tips and rationale, 21–27
    urgent care, 95–96
triage acuity scales, 69–74
    Australasian Triage Scale, 72–73
    Canadian Triage and Acuity Scale, 70, 72
    Emergency Severity Index, 70, 72
    Manchester Triage System, 73
    overview of, 69–70
triage competency, 33
    case scenario/case study packets, 35
    components of, 35–36
    education vs. competency, 33–34
    feedback, 35
        exemplars, 35
        posttests, 35
    methods of evaluating, 34–35

observation, 34
retrospective chart review, 34–35, 36–37
audit form, 273
by others, 37
for self-review, 36–37
Triage Competency Validation form, 269–270
Triage Education and Competency Plan, 271
triage nurse, 4–5
and charge nurse/patient flow coordinator, communication between, 104
courses and certifications, 5
personal awareness for, 29–32
qualifications of, 4–5
roles of, 41–42
techniques to keep safe, 238
triage nursing
customer experience in, 49–57
legal concerns in, 59–64
triage orientation, 7–10
communication, 8–9
completion of, 9–10, 17–18
equipment lists, 9
evaluation techniques, 17
policies and procedures, 16
purpose of
current knowledge, advancing, 6
documentation skills, enhancing, 6
policies and procedures, understanding, 7
"red flag" patient presentations, identifying, 7
triage flow, understanding, 6
triage role, understanding, 6
resources for, 10, 16
right preceptors for, selecting, 8
skills and processes, 16–17
teamwork, 9
triage preceptor
qualifications of, 15
traits of, 15
triage staff
and other departments, communication between, 104
and patients/support systems, communication between, 104–105
role of, 102–103
Triage Tip Binder/Triage Tip Electronic Folder, 27
tuberculosis, 130

urgent care centers (UCCs), 93–96
background of, 93–94
regulations for, 94
service and scope, 95
staffing at, 94
triage, role of, 95–96

vaginal bleeding, 116
verbal abuse, 233
verbal violence, 31
veterans, 13, 14
victims of violence, 192
violence
active, 255–262
intimate partner violence, 203–204
lateral, 31–32
consequences of, 31
prevention of, 31–32
physical, 31
potential for, 234–236
psychological, 31
types of, 233–234
verbal, 31
victims of, 192
visually impaired patient, 207–208
vital signs, 121
abdominal emergencies, 147
pediatric triage, 215

waiting room (WR)
crowded, 234–236, 237
discharging patients from, 107
benefits of, 108

waiting room (WR) (*cont.*)
    challenges of, 107–108
    rapid triage assessment, 42–43
    rounding, 55
weapon concealment, 258
weapon palming, 258
whooping cough, 129
Women Escaping a Violent Environment (WEAVE), 244
worst-case scenarios, 122
    abdominal emergencies, 146
    behavioral health emergencies, 162
    cardiac emergencies, 134
    endocrine emergencies, 177
    environmental emergencies, 182
    musculoskeletal emergencies, 174
    neurological emergencies, 140
    obstetric and gynecological emergencies, 154
    ocular emergencies, 168
    red flag patient presentations, 122
    respiratory emergencies, 126
    trauma emergencies, 188

FAST FACTS FOR YOUR NURSING CAREER

Choose from Over 40 Titles!

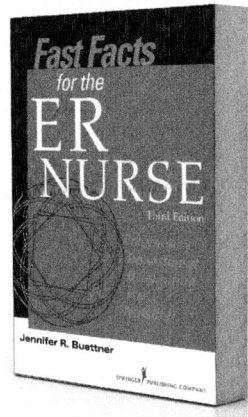
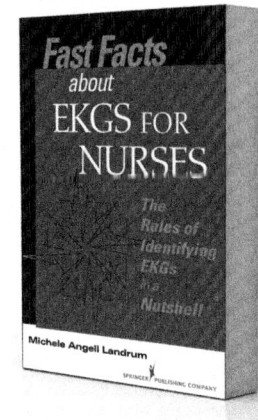
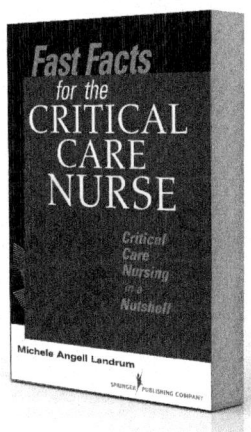
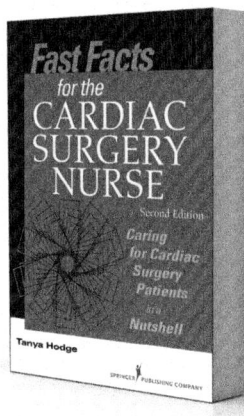

These must-have reference books are packed with timely, useful, and accessible information presented in a clear, precise format. Pocket-sized and affordable, the series provides quick access to information you need to know and use daily.

springerpub.com/FastFacts

NWTC Library
2740 W. Mason St.
Green Bay, WI 54307